ASTHMA
at your fingertips

'. . . A helpful and clearly written book . . .'

Dr Martyn Partridge, Chief Medical Advisor, National Asthma Campaign

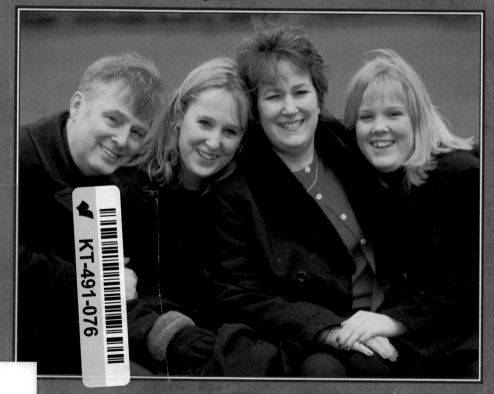

THIRD EDITION

Dr Mark Levy
Professor Sean Hilton • Greta Barnes MBE

Comments on **Asthma at your fingertips** *from readers*

"Having asthma should not stop you leading a full and active life. With knowledge of my condition, the correct treatment and a desire to succeed, I became the Olympic champion.

This book gives you the knowledge. Don't limit yourself."

Adrian Moorhouse, MBE, Olympic Gold Medallist

"This book provides the information necessary for those with asthma (and for those who live with those with asthma) to take control of their condition."

Dr Martyn Partridge, Chief Medical Adviser,
National Asthma Campaign

"This book is essential reading for both people with asthma and their doctors. It is easy to understand, and clearly and simply explains the different treatments now available for asthma.

Asthma sufferers and anyone involved in their care will find it of great benefit."

Dr Caroline Sykes, General Practitioner, London

"I had the book bought as a Christmas present and I could not put it down. If I was not reading it my Dad was. Along with good pictures and clear information I really felt that somebody out there was listening to what asthmatics go through.

The book has given me great confidence and I feel that I am able to do more things than before."

Mrs Debbie Clarke, Birmingham

"Your book was a pleasure to read: a clear, concise, informative account of the causes, symptoms, treatment and partial prevention of asthmatic conditions. I am glad I chose it amongst all the others available."

A. Roberts, Surrey

"It is the best book I have read on asthma and the medication required to control it. Certainly a lot of research had gone into writing the book and I would like you to pass on our best wishes to the authors involved."

Janice Fairbridge, Middlesborough

"I am pleased to be able to recommend it highly for patients with asthma and all who are involved in their care."

Professor E.D. Bateman, Respiratory Clinic,
Groote Schuur Hospital, South Africa

Comments on **Asthma at your fingertips** *from readers (continued)*

"...splendidly helpful."

Daphne Lutley, Devon

"...I devoured your book."

C. Thornberry, South Africa

"I have learnt so much more from your book than I have from the medical profession. You have changed my attitude towards my asthma, to look at it as taking control over it and not letting it dominate my life."

Mrs Penny Alderwick, Bristol

"It certainly contains a lot of information which will undoubtedly help patients understand and cope with their disease. I shall be more than happy to recommend this book."

Dr Michael Rudolf, Consultant Physician, Ealing Hospital NHS Trust

"The authors are to be congratulated for making a very complex situation very understandable."

Professor Clive Page, Biomedical Sciences Division, King's College London

"I think it is an excellent book and one that will be very helpful."

Professor Richard Beasley, Professor of Medicine, Wellington School of Medicine, New Zealand

"Answers in a clear and readily understood fashion the questions that my patients ask and need information on. The format is simple and accessible."

Dr David Bellamy, General Practitioner, Bournemouth

"An important contribution for asthma sufferers. It also provides support for health professionals."

Dr M.D.L. Morgan, Glenfield Hospital NHS Trust, Leicester

"Extremely helpful, simply and well written."

Dr G. Skadding, Consultant Physician, Royal National Throat Nose and Ear Hospital

Reviews of **Asthma at your fingertips**

"**Asthma at your fingertips** explains what causes asthma and gives a detailed explanation of the treatments available, guiding the reader through the complex world of inhalers, steroids and asthma clinics. The book devotes a whole chapter to children – from giving inhalers to babies to how best a child can cope at school – as well as looking at the way asthma can affect different areas of life, from pregnancy to work and even sex."

Essentials

"This is a brilliant little book that has been written by experts in the management of asthma in primary care. The authors include two general practitioners, and Greta Barnes – a specialist asthma nurse who runs the National Asthma and Respiratory Training Centre.

The book is written as a self-care manual, divided into sections such as what is asthma, issues to do with treatment, monitoring, coping in everyday life, and in emergencies, the needs of children, self help and complementary therapies. The book is organised around questions and answers. The success of this technique is in its clarity. The authors have provided enough information at a level that avoids being patronising. Surprisingly enough it is also very readable and avoids jargon and dense or medical writing. There is a sensitivity, but also an honesty about the limits of professional knowledge. There is a very useful glossary and index and list of addresses."

District Nursing Association Newsletter

"This new publication on asthma is undoubtedly excellent value for money, particularly for those who suffer from asthma or for parents of children who are affected.

Despite the book being aimed at this audience, it certainly has a place in the nursing and medical libraries, to complement the wealth of literature on the subject.

The book is logically presented and amusingly illustrated with cartoons. Clear diagrams are incorporated into the text and supported by colour plates. Information has been provided largely on a 'question and answer' basis, applying technical terminology which has been consistently and coherently explained. Chapters are also included on non-medical treatments and self help groups for people with asthma. Essentially, this is a comprehensive and practical guide to prevention, control and treatment of asthma which would be beneficial to sufferers, families, nurses and doctors."

Nursing Standard

Reviews of **Asthma at your fingertips** *(continued)*

"I feel that this book is a great step forward in giving information to clients and is an essential reference for all health centres and public libraries. Even I, as someone who knows about and lives with the disease, picked up a few helpful ideas from this book and can highly recommend it to anyone involved in patient education about asthma and for those who suffer with asthma."

Nursing Times

"This book will be welcomed by asthmatics, their relatives, and the many health professionals who are often asked to recommend a book.

The authors are to be congratulated on the comprehensive contents, clear layout and the ease with which the book can be used...

This book is well thought out and has been put together with the utmost care. It is a very useful addition to any asthmatic's and health professional's bookshelf."

Practice Nursing

"Although most general practitioners will only learn a little from this book, I doubt there will be any general practitioner who will learn nothing. It is of special interest to those running asthma clinics, their nurses and patients."

Therapeutics Update

"This book may be considered one of the most valuable, comprehensive and readable of its kind. It is highly recommended for all patients who can be persuaded to learn more about their illness and embark on a programme of self management. All who care for patients with asthma are also advised to have one on their shelves."

South African Medical Journal

"This [book] benefits from being presented in a question-and-answer format and offers an excellent judgement on all the things you had meant to ask your GP but never got round to."

Asthma News

Asthma at your fingertips

THE COMPREHENSIVE AND MEDICALLY ACCURATE MANUAL ON HOW TO MANAGE YOUR ASTHMA

THIRD EDITION

Mark Levy MBChB, FRCGP
General Practitioner, Kenton, Middlesex; Editor, Asthma in General Practice; *Secretary, General Practice and Primary Care Group (European Respiratory Society)*

Sean Hilton MD, FRCGP
General Practitioner, Kingston upon Thames, and Professor of General Practice, St George's Hospital Medical School, London

Greta Barnes MBE, SRN
Director, The National Asthma and Respiratory Training Centre, Warwick, and Member of the National Asthma Task Force

CLASS PUBLISHING · LONDON

Printing history
First published 1993
Reprinted 1993, 1994
Revised edition 1994
Reprinted 1996
Second edition 1997
Reprinted 1997
Third edition 2000

The rights of Mark Levy, Sean Hilton and Greta Barnes to be identified as the authors of this work have been asserted by them in accordance with the Copyright, Designs and Patents Act 1988

The information presented in this book is accurate and current to the best of the author's knowledge. The author and publisher, however, make no guarantee as to, and assume no responsibility for, the correctness, sufficiency or completeness of such information or recommendation. The reader is advised to consult a doctor regarding all aspects of individual health care.

Products mentioned in the text are trademarks of the manufacturers listed in the Appendix and Table B in the Colour Plate Section. In particular, the following products are trademarks of the GlaxoWellcome group of companies: Becloforte, Becotide, Flixotide, Seretide, Serevent, Ventide, Ventolin; Accuhaler, Diskhaler, Easi-Breathe, Evohaler, Rotahaler; Babyhaler, Integra, Volumatic.

The authors and publishers welcome feedback from the users of this book. Please contact the publishers.

Class Publishing, Barb House, Barb Mews, London W6 7PA, UK
Telephone: (020) 7371 2119
Fax: (020) 7371 2878
email: post@class.co.uk

A CIP catalogue record for this book is available from the British Library

ISBN 1 85959 006 3

Designed by Wendy Bann
Cartoons by Paul Davies
Illustrations by David Woodroffe
Edited by Michèle Clarke
Indexed by Val Elliston
Production by Landmark Production Consultants Ltd, Princes Risborough
Typesetting by DP Photosetting, Aylesbury, Bucks
Printed and bound in Finland by WS Bookwell, Juva

Contents

DEDICATION
To our families

Acknowledgements

We would like to thank all those practice nurses who took the time to ask their patients for questions on asthma.

We are indebted to those people with asthma who kindly provided us with the genuine questions used in this book.

We are grateful to Roberta Williams for her innovative ideas, to the late John Donaldson, and Sue Rout for reading the manuscript and making useful comments on it.

We would like to thank the National Asthma and Respiratory Training Centre for providing line illustrations of devices.

We thank the companies who kindly provided colour illustrations: Allen & Hanburys Ltd, Clement Clarke International Ltd, Celltech Medeva and 3M Health Care Ltd.

The text for the answer to the question 'Are there any occupations I will have to avoid?' on page 143 was modified from *Asthma* by Clark, Godfrey and Lee by kind permission of the publishers, Chapman and Hall.

Foreword

by Dr Martyn R. Partridge MD, FRCP

Chief Medical Adviser to the National Asthma Campaign, and Consultant Chest Physician, Whipps Cross Hospital, London

As a result of research performed in the UK and abroad, our understanding of what causes asthma, what is happening in the airways of those with asthma and how best we treat the condition has advanced considerably over the last few years.

Within the next decade we may have enough knowledge of what causes the condition to be able to give meaningful advice to mothers-to-be about actions they can take to reduce the chances of their offspring developing asthma. Until that time is reached, we need to ensure that all of those with this common condition benefit maximally from that which is available. Recent research has given us a clearer idea of how best to deliver care to those with asthma and has provided evidence of the advantages of giving control of the condition to the person with asthma, with guidance from their health professionals.

This book provides the information necessary for those with asthma (and for those who live with those with asthma) to take control of their condition. The authors are at the forefront of delivery of care to those with asthma and have considerable experience in the field of education. We should be grateful to them for producing such a helpul and clearly written book.

Introduction

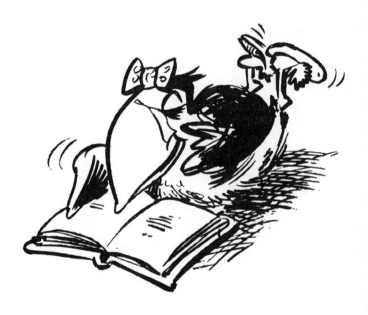

If you have asthma, or if you are a relative or close friend of someone who has asthma, we hope that you will find this book helpful. Our aim is to provide you with information and practical tips which will enable you to manage your asthma, reduce the problems it produces for you, and to lead a life which is not restricted by it. This may appear ambitious, but there is no doubt that it is people with asthma and their families who have the main responsibility for day to day care. We believe that it is vital for you to be involved in your own care (that is in 'self-care' or 'self-management') as you are the person who lives with the asthma day in and day out.

What this book is not	*What this book is*
1 A medical textbook	1 Questions of importance for anyone interested in asthma
2 A list of asthma terms	2 Clear answers to questions and problems (where they can be given!)
3 A history of asthma	3 Descriptions of the condition we call asthma, as we understand it today
4 A collection of our favourite cases with asthma	4 Practical questions asked by people
5 A reference book for research studies	5 Practical help (based on research findings) that makes living with asthma easier
6 A list of cures and possible cures	6 Information about asthma management – what is effective, what is available, what may become available in the future

In 1995, representatives of the medical profession in the UK produced guidelines for the management of asthma. They stated that the aims of management should be as shown in the box.

AIMS OF MANAGEMENT
- to recognize asthma
- to abolish symptoms
- to restore normal or best possible long-term airway function
- to reduce the risk of severe attack
- to enable normal growth in children
- to minimize absence from school or work

However mild your asthma may be, we believe there are certain basic principles and skills with which you should be familiar. As well as these, this book contains more detailed information for anyone with more complex asthma, or who may have had asthma for many years and have more 'advanced' questions to pose.

Inevitably some of the terms we use are medical or technical. We have tried to explain these terms wherever they occur, and have attempted to steer clear of medical jargon. We have also included a glossary of some of the more important (and perhaps confusing) medical terms that tend to crop up time and again. When these terms appear in the text for the first time, they are in *italic* type.

When it comes to drugs used in the treatment of asthma, we have tried to be consistent in the names we have used. There are many brand names for anti-asthma drugs, as well as the true (or generic) names. Where a particular name has been included in the question we have continued to use that name. You will find more detail about our use of drug names in the introduction to the chapter on **Treatment**.

Throughout the book you will find frequent references to peak flow meters and peak expiratory flow readings. The peak flow meter is a small and simple piece of equipment that can measure, on a scale, how hard you can blow. When your airways are narrowed, as during an asthma attack, the reading you get on the scale will be reduced. When you are well, the reading will be higher. It is as simple as that. We feel that monitoring the peak expiratory flow combined with recognizing the presence of symptoms is the best way to follow the course of your asthma (rather like using a blood pressure machine to follow blood pressure). This does not mean that we believe everyone with asthma should be using peak flow meters **all the time** to monitor their asthma, but when problems arise they do give the best assessment of how severe the asthma is. In the book we refer to readings which either are a percentage of what you should be able to blow (e.g. 50% of your best reading) or actual readings (e.g. 400 *litres per minute*). These are the units used to measure peak flow, and in this example your lungs have the power to blow 400 litres of air per minute out through your mouth. There is an entire section in Chapter 3 devoted to peak flow readings, and how to use them. At the present time there is no cure for asthma, and no immediate prospect of one. Thrilling developments in genetics and cell biology are revealing more and more about how it is we develop asthma, and just what goes wrong at the level of the cells. Once we have a full understanding of these processes, the search for a cure will surely be successful. In the meantime, there is much we can do to improve the application of the knowledge we already have about asthma. Many people are suffering unnecessarily either because they are not receiving the right treatment, or because they do not realize the benefits of effective treatment.

How to use this book

Because different people have very different requirements for information about asthma, this book has been designed in a way that means you do not have to read it from cover to cover. The questions are arranged into chapters and sections, so you may care to dip into the book in sections at a time, or look for the answer to a particular question by using the contents table and the index.

If you have just been diagnosed as having asthma, we suggest that you concentrate on the following sections first: *Symptoms* and *Triggers* in Chapter 1; *Drug treatments* and *Devices* in Chapter 2; and *Recognising uncontrolled asthma* in Chapter 3. If you are more experienced in managing your own asthma, you may wish to concentrate more on the *Peak flow monitoring* section in Chapter 3 and on Chapters 4 and 6. If your child has asthma, we hope that Chapter 5 will deal with many of your concerns. Chapter 7 is devoted to non-drug methods of approaching asthma management.

This style means that inevitably there will be some repetition within the book, and a few questions that appear to be duplicated in different sections. There is some cross referencing of questions, but we have tried to keep this to a minimum. We would prefer each question to be answered in full, rather than direct you to a number of different sections each time, but for reasons of space this is not always possible.

This book has been assembled from real questions that we have been asked by hundreds of real people with real asthma! Not everyone will agree that the questions we have chosen are the important ones, and certainly not everyone will agree with the answers we have provided. Future editions of this book can be improved by feedback from the people who know most about problems relating to asthma – in other words, you. If you have any comments about the contents of the book we would be delighted to receive them. Please write to us, c/o Class Publishing, Barb House, Barb Mews, London W6 7PA, UK.

What is Asthma?

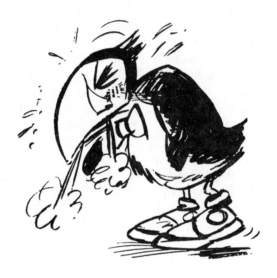

Introduction

During the last 50 years, asthma has become recognized as one of the most important medical conditions in the Western World. In the UK today there are nearly three million sufferers in all, and nearly half of these are children. Indeed asthma is the commonest chronic condition affecting children and at least one in 10 of all children, and probably more, suffer from it at any one time.

There is a wide spectrum of severity in asthma in both adults and children. Many are at the mild end of the range, with only occasional problems and a limited need for treatments. A few have very severe asthma, with repeated admissions to hospital, and a life that is extremely restricted by their asthma. However, the majority of people with asthma can realistically hope and expect to lead full lives, free from symptoms, if their condition is well managed.

It has been estimated that in 1996 the cost of asthma to the economy of the UK approached two billion pounds. This cost was borne by the National Health Service, the Department of Social Security (in invalidity payments), and by lost productivity. There are few conditions with greater impact than this.

When you are first told that you have asthma, many thoughts will flash through your mind. If you have a close friend or relative with the condition, inevitably you will wonder whether your own asthma will be like theirs. We state repeatedly throughout this book (and we make no apology for doing so) that asthma is an extremely variable condition. No two people have the same pattern of symptoms, and even for the same person symptoms may vary dramatically at different times. The key is to get to know your own asthma as well as you can, and not to be too influenced by what happens to other people.

Having said that, we propose to spend this first chapter dealing with general questions about the nature of asthma. This involves some anatomy and physiology (i.e. the structure of the body and how it works), but we have tried to keep this straightforward and relevant. Because it varies so much, many people assume that there must be many types of asthma. This is not so, but the section *Is it really asthma and is there more than one type?* deals with some of these questions.

The most basic question of all – *What is asthma?* – comes first. After this there comes a section on symptoms of asthma. This also explains what causes the symptoms, so that we can understand why and how they arise. The section on *Triggers* covers most of the important factors that may spark off attacks of asthma, or episodes of increased symptoms. Other sections deal with the questions we have frequently been asked about inheritance of asthma and whether or not it is all in the mind.

Asthma explained

What is asthma?

Asthma (full name bronchial asthma) is a condition which causes difficulty in moving air into and out of the *lungs* as we breathe. The lungs (see Figure 1.1) are the organs of breathing and are often described as being like a pair of large sponges. They do look like sponges, but in terms of their structure and function it is easier to think of the lungs as an upside down tree. You breathe air in through the trunk (the main windpipe, or *trachea*); it travels though the larger branches and then the smaller branches and twigs (the airways, or *bronchi*) until it reaches the leaves (the air spaces, or *alveoli*). It is in the air spaces that the oxygen passes from the air into the bloodstream. Carbon dioxide is passed out in the opposite direction.

If you have asthma, you have a problem with your *airways*, or bronchi. They become narrowed, making it more difficult for air to

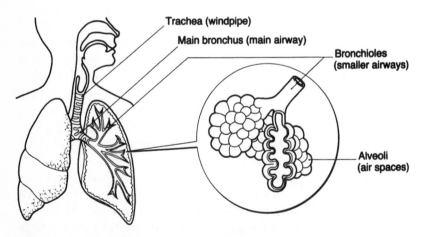

Figure 1.1 This diagram shows what the lungs look like inside. Breathed air goes from the windpipe (trachea) into the two main airways (bronchi). From there it goes through the small bronchioles to the air spaces (alveoli) and then is absorbed into the bloodstream.

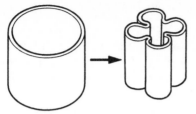

1   Tightening of airways from muscle spasm with reduced space

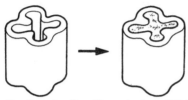

2   Swelling of walls, with production of thick mucus

Figure 1.2   In asthma the airways narrow due to spasm (tightening) of the muscles around them and swelling of the lining and sticky mucus inside them.

move to and from the air spaces. The underlying reason for this narrowing is an *inflammation* of the lining of your airways. This inflammation has several effects. It makes your airways very twitchy, or irritable, so that your response to any form of irritation or stimulus is coughing, and a tightening of the muscles that surround the airways. It also makes the lining of your airways swollen, and may cause you to produce lots of sticky mucus or phlegm.

The result of all this is that the bore, or diameter, of your airways is reduced in three ways: spasm (tightening) of muscles around it; swelling of the lining itself; and production of sticky mucus which tends to block it (see Figure 1.2).

(There is another condition, sometimes called *cardiac asthma*, which is quite different from this. Cardiac asthma is a rather old fashioned term to describe acute heart failure, and most doctors now do not use it. It has nothing in common with bronchial asthma except that it causes difficulty in breathing.)

Am I right in believing that asthma is caused by a reduction in size of the airways?

You are right in believing this. The underlying problem in asthma is an inflammation of the lining of the airways. This makes the airways irritable (causing a cough) and also narrows the airways in three different ways. Firstly, the inflammation causes spasm (tightening) of the muscles surrounding the airways; secondly the lining itself becomes swollen; and thirdly excess sticky mucus is produced. All these lead to a reduction in the size (width) of the airways (see Figure 1.2), causing wheezing and shortness of breath.

So, to be strictly accurate, asthma causes a reduction in the size of the airways, and that produces the symptoms.

Is asthma a virus?

No, asthma is not a virus, it is a condition which results from an inflammation of the airways. A *virus* is a germ, an infectious agent, that invades human cells and causes illness. There are thousands of different types of viruses. They cause illness of all sorts, from the common cold, measles, to hepatitis and many others. There is, though, an important link between asthma and viruses. The link is that the most common asthma *trigger* of all is an *upper respiratory tract infection* (common cold) caused by a virus. A class of virus known as the *rhinoviruses* is most often responsible, but there are others that can do it, including the virus responsible for influenza.

So when you have a cold which 'goes to your chest' and makes your asthma worse, remember that it is a virus infection that is attacking you. Viruses do not get better with antibiotics, so your first move should be to increase your asthma therapy, and not to rush for antibiotics.

Is my asthma an allergy?

Asthma and *allergy* are not the same, but asthma can be triggered by an *allergic reaction* to substances such as grass pollen, house dust mite and pet hair. If you have an allergy, it means that you are sensitive to ordinary everyday substances to which most people do not react. For example, most people sneeze if pepper gets into their nose, and everyone's eyes will water if they peel onions. People with allergies will react in similar ways (getting itchy eyes, a runny nose or wheezing) if they come into contact with something to which they are allergic. For those allergic to cats, handling, stroking, or even being in the same room as one will produce these symptoms.

Generally speaking an allergy develops over a long time and an allergic reaction does not happen the first time you come into contact with a substance. Some people's asthma is certainly triggered by an allergy. If you are one of these people and if the *allergen* can be found then it would be sensible to avoid or reduce the amount of contact with the offending substance wherever possible. However, this may be easier said than done!

Is asthma catching? For example, can I give it to my daughter?

To say something is 'catching' is usually taken to mean that it is an infectious disease. To this we can answer with certainty – no, asthma cannot be 'caught' from someone who has it, as one catches a cold. The condition does tend to run in families and because of this people may tend to believe that it is an infectious disease. Asthma appears to be more common now and this may also lead to the false impression that the disease is 'spreading' like an infectious disease.

How did my asthma start – and why?

Without knowing all the details of your *medical history*, we cannot say how or why you have asthma, but we can give you some idea about what is currently known about the causes of asthma.

The tendency to start asthma is something that is inherited by a proportion of the population. It is called a 'genetic predisposition' and is described in more detail in the section on ***Inheritance*** later in this chapter. However, as with many other conditions, it is a combination of genetic and environmental factors that leads to actual symptoms. We are beginning to understand more about the factors that convert the airways into their 'twitchy' state. The correct term for this twitchiness is *bronchial hyperreactivity*

(BHR). This means, simply, bronchi that overreact. In children it may be a single virus infection (e.g. a cold), or many respiratory infections during a critical period that unmask the symptoms.

Increasing evidence points to an important role for allergy as another important factor in the environment in which we live. We now know that mothers who smoke during pregnancy have babies who are more likely to develop harmful allergy antibodies (substances produced by the *immune system*). Meeting substances to which we might be allergic (such as pets, or high house dust mite levels) early in life may switch on BHR, leading to childhood asthma. Some similar process may take place in adults.

An equally fascinating question – as yet unanswered – is why does asthma appear to stop? Many people lose their asthma symptoms, for no obvious reason, for periods of months or years. We now think of this as people going into remission rather than people outgrowing asthma. If we knew why they do this, it would help us to explain how asthma starts.

Can asthma be cured?

No. Although enormous advances have been made in the treatment and management of asthma there is unfortunately no cure, as yet. However, gene therapy is a future possibility.

Because of the nature of the condition there are times when people feel they must be cured because they are completely without symptoms. Whilst this symptomless state (called *remission*) can go on for months and even years it has to be remembered that once you have had asthma you will always have the tendency to have it again, and therefore you are at some degree of risk. It is probably better to think of asthma going into remission rather than being cured.

Symptoms

What are the symptoms?

The main symptoms of asthma are coughing, wheezing and shortness of breath: **coughing** occurs because the airways are irritable and twitchy from their inflamed lining; **wheezing**, because of the air whistling through narrowed airways makes a high pitched noise; and **shortness of breath** because the body has to work harder than usual to carry out the normal process of breathing. There are other symptoms, such as a feeling of tightness in the chest, or sharp chest pains, and some which are less common, such as tingling or itching of the skin.

Why do I usually not wheeze when I have asthma – my chest just feels tight?

Wheezing is only one of the symptoms of asthma – some people never wheeze. The other main symptoms are coughing and shortness of breath. Chest tightness, such as you describe, is another common symptom. Asthma causes narrowing of the airways in three ways: mucus (phlegm) inside the airways; thickening (swelling) of the walls of the airways; and muscle contraction (tightening) in the walls of the airways (see Figure 1.2). This narrowing of the airways can cause wheezing, but much depends on the level of the narrowing – there may be no wheeze if it is slight. Very often in mild asthma there is just a persistent dry cough, or some shortness of breath.

There is an entirely different situation in asthma where there may be no wheeze. During an *acute* attack, if your airways are very tight and air cannot get into or out of your lungs, you will not wheeze. This is known as a 'silent chest'. It is very dangerous and urgent medical attention is required. Someone in this situation may look blue (look at the tongue) indicating that the blood is not carrying enough oxygen.

As asthma is a lung condition, why is it that my throat seems to close, so that I feel as if I'm being strangled?

Your lungs contain thousands of air passages which range in size from the main windpipe (trachea) starting in the throat to the smallest airways, the bronchioles, which empty into the air spaces, the alveoli (see Figure 1.1). Asthma affects all of these air passages to some degree. In the majority of people it is the smaller air passages deep inside the lungs that are most affected. However, in some people – like you – it affects mainly the larger ones, even up to the trachea, and this is why you have a sensation of being strangled during an attack. Not only is this very unpleasant for you, but it tends to be slower to respond to treatment than the more common form.

My son has experienced a rash while suffering an asthmatic cough. Is this rare, and are the two connected?

People do occasionally complain of itching when they have a flare up of their asthma. However, we are not aware of any relationship between an asthmatic cough and a rash. There may be several explanations, but one of the commonest complications of any treatment with drugs is a skin reaction. Whilst exact figures are difficult to obtain, it is known that approximately 3% of all patients taking medicines will develop a drug-related rash. If your son was taking a different treatment for his cough at the time the rash developed, then the drug could be the cause, rather than his asthma. Some respiratory infections (which often provoke asthma) are also known to cause a temporary rash. This is parti-cularly true of viral chest infections (similar to the common cold) in children.

Another possibility is that your son has *atopic eczema*. This is a skin inflammation which occurs in people who have an inherited tendency towards allergic problems. It often coexists with other allergic conditions, especially asthma and *hay fever*. It is not uncommon for eczema to flare up at the same time as an episode of asthma.

Does vomiting set off attacks of asthma in children?

Vomiting is one of the more unusual symptoms of asthma, but a minority of people get it whenever they suffer an uncontrolled asthma episode. This may also happen in adults, but is more common in children. A cold often sparks off the attack, and this is followed by episodes of vomiting which may last for days. The vomit contains amounts of mucus (slimy phlegm). The vomiting may be so severe that a child can become *dehydrated* (short of fluid) and even need hospital admission. Eventually, the chest tightness eases, and recovery occurs gradually.

It can be the other way round sometimes, so that the asthma

sets off the vomiting. Pressure from distended lungs and coughing may push down on the diaphragm, and squeeze the stomach, leading to vomiting. In these cases children often improve greatly after they have vomited, probably because there is less pressure on the diaphragm.

What causes the chest pain I get when my asthma is bad?

There are three main causes of chest pain during uncontrolled asthma. These all occur as a result of stretching in the chest, and any or all of them may be the cause of your pain.

- During an asthma attack the lungs expand greatly, because a lot of air becomes trapped in them. The *pleurae* (which are membranes surrounding the lungs) stretch as a result, and this may cause pain.
- The walls of the chest also stretch due to the overexpansion of the lungs. This causes strain on the rib joints (where the ribs join the breastbone, and at the back where they join the spine). This can also cause pain.
- The muscles between the ribs are also stretched when the lungs are overexpanded, and this may be a third cause of the pain.

Many people think automatically about their hearts and heart attacks when chest pain is mentioned. Chest pain during asthma episodes rarely comes from the heart, unless it occurs in those people with known heart disease.

Why do I have so little energy when my asthma is bad?

There may be a few reasons why you feel weak or lack energy when your asthma is bad. The main job for the lungs is to help oxygen get from the air to the blood (they also help to remove waste products like carbon dioxide from the body). Oxygen is needed by the vital organs of the body, e.g. the heart, brain and kidneys. When the body is short of oxygen the vital organs get tired and you feel short of energy. When your asthma is bad your airways become narrowed, oxygen cannot get through, and this leads to your lack of energy. A virus infection (e.g. a cold) is the commonest trigger for asthma and the virus itself often makes people feel tired.

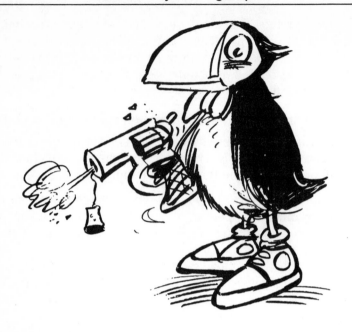

Triggers

What triggers asthma symptoms?

Triggers do **not** cause asthma – they are factors which **may** bring on symptoms or attacks of asthma. There are seven main triggers.

1 **Virus infections of the upper respiratory tract** (mainly colds or 'flu). Everyone with asthma will be familiar with the cold that 'goes to the chest'. Overall, this is the commonest trigger for episodes of asthma, particularly in young children, and accounts for the peak in asthma attacks that occurs in the autumn, when colds are rife.
2 **Exercise**. All forms of *exercise*, but particularly running, can bring on asthma symptoms within a few minutes. Treatment is usually effective in preventing this sort of asthma.
3 **Emotional factors and stress**. Overexcitement in children and laughter are perhaps the two emotions most likely to bring

on symptoms. Stress may bring on asthma attacks, or make symptoms worse.

4 **Atmospheric conditions**. Changes in weather and temperature are well known to provoke symptoms. In the UK, cold dry air is perhaps the best example (in Hong Kong, by contrast, the rainy season is known to be the peak time for asthma). Other atmospheres, not necessarily weather related, can also make asthma worse, for example those in pubs or clubs. The polluted atmospheres of inner urban areas are also important triggers of asthma symptoms.

5 **Cigarette smoke**.

6 **Allergies**. For many people allergies are the most important triggers for their asthma symptoms or attacks, even more than colds and other virus infections. The substance causing the allergy is known as the allergen. The most important allergen in the UK is the *house dust mite*, a microscopic insect which inhabits our home environment in millions, living on scales of dead human skin. The other major allergens responsible for asthma are house dust itself; feathers; animal fur or hair (*danders*), particularly from dogs, cats and horses; grass and tree pollens; and mould spores. People who have seasonal rhinitis (hay fever, allergy to pollen) may find that their asthma gets worse when the pollen counts are high. Therefore, appropriate treatment of the pollen allergy helps to prevent and treat asthma episodes. One particularly important type of allergy is the sensitivity that can develop to substances in the work environment.

7 **Drugs**. We know that certain drugs can cause asthma in some people. Most important of these is aspirin, because it is a drug which is available without prescription, and is taken by most of the adult population. In a small proportion (1–2%) of adults with asthma, aspirin can cause serious, even life-threatening attacks. *Non-steroidal anti-inflammatory drugs* (*NSAIDS* like Nurofen, ibuprofen) can make asthma worse, particularly in people with *nasal polyps*. Another group of drugs to avoid is the *beta blockers*, commonly used to treat high blood pressure and heart problems. If you do have these problems as well as asthma there are plenty of alternative, effective drugs that you can take quite safely.

How can I find out what triggers my asthma if the cause is not obvious?

We have listed the common trigger factors for asthma symptoms in the first question of this section. However, it is not always easy for you to find out what the most important trigger for your asthma is. One reason for this is that the reaction to a trigger may

Date									
Symptoms									
Cough									
Wheeze									
Shortness of breath									
Peak flow									
650									
600									
300									
100									
50									
Worked today									
Exercised today									
Decorated the house									
Cleaned house									
Worked with dust									
Worked in garden									
Caught cold									
Tried a different food									

Figure 1.3   Daily symptom diary chart

come after many hours (known as the *late reaction*), rather than immediately. This makes it more difficult to spot the connection between your coming into contact with a trigger, and your asthma.

A daily symptom diary chart is an ideal way for you to find out about your particular triggers. The peak flow charts used for self-management are available from your doctor, and these may be helpful. However, it may be best to draw a chart specially marked with possible triggers for your own particular situation. This can be done by taking a page of graph paper and marking it as shown in Figure 1.3.

These of course are only a few of the possible trigger factors. Others may be added to this list, as and when you suspect them. For example if you go horse riding occasionally, add this to your chart, and follow your symptoms for 24 hours or more afterwards. By marking your chart daily, using a 'Y' for yes when you have come up against the possible trigger and comparing it with your asthma symptoms, it may be possible to identify a pattern. It is not always obvious from a peak flow chart which triggers have been responsible; symptoms may be more helpful. It may be necessary for you to do some calculations on your daily peak flow readings to check if they have in fact changed. You will find more information about taking peak flow readings and keeping charts in Chapter 3.

Having given you all this information, we have to admit that for some people, particularly those whose asthma starts in adulthood, it may prove impossible to find a clearly identifiable trigger, and you are left needing to control your asthma as effectively as possible with treatment.

Do different substances (triggers) affect different people?

Yes, but most people with asthma respond to a small number of common trigger factors. Everyone's airways (including people who do not suffer from asthma) will react to certain inhaled irritants. For example, people cough when they go into a smoky room or when a crumb goes down the wrong way.

People who suffer from allergic asthma (also called *extrinsic asthma*) overreact to particular types of allergen – usually well recognized substances. These are called specific allergens. The most important ones are house dust mite, grass pollens and animal fur or hair, but there are many others. Particular allergens may trigger off a dramatic narrowing of the airways in someone with allergic asthma.

Other people with asthma respond to different triggers such as virus infections, fumes, air pollution, exercise, cold air and laughter. These triggers are not allergens. If these people are not affected by the specific allergies listed above, they are said to have *intrinsic asthma*. Often they are people who develop asthma later in life, and who are not 'allergic'. However, there are many unfortunate people who fall into both 'camps', and whose asthma is triggered by both specific allergens and non-specific triggers.

This can all seem very confusing! It emphasizes the importance of anyone with asthma knowing which triggers – if any – are important in their own individual case.

Why should the smell from a wood shop or a sawmill start off my attacks?

Wood dust is a trigger for asthma in some people, and you may be one of them. It is usually the fine wood dust found in sawmills or in industrial wood cutting, rather than the coarse sawdust associated with general building work. It is not the smell which starts off your attack, but the fine dust. If you are close enough to smell the wood, you are close enough to inhale the dust.

Why is my asthma worse at night?

Nobody knows for sure the answer to this question. It is fair to say that most things **seem** to be worse at night – from toothache to anxiety or loneliness. However, with asthma, problems really **are** worse at night.

Many things in your body vary from day to night. For example, some blood hormones and chemicals have higher blood levels during the day than in the night. You will see a similar pattern with your *peak expiratory flow* (PEF) – readings are usually low in the night and early mornings and higher in the evenings. There are many explanations for this variation but none has yet been totally convincing. The better controlled your asthma is, the less likely are troublesome night time problems going to be.

Morning to evening difference in peak flow (called the *diurnal*

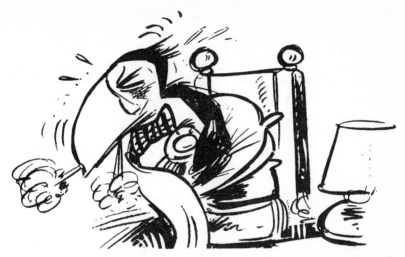

variation) is a good measure of how well controlled your asthma is. Normally, this variation should be less than 15%. Differences greater than this suggest poorly controlled asthma. If you are taking treatment but having frequent night-time symptoms, you should discuss this with your doctor or asthma nurse. They may be able to suggest changes to your treatment plan that will help to improve your control.

Why does the cold weather make me wheeze?

Breathing in cold air often makes people wheeze and cough, and can sometimes trigger off dramatic asthma symptoms. This is more likely to happen if the air is dry as well as cold. Cold air is one of the inhaled irritants which can make your airways 'twitchy'. This tendency to twitchiness is called bronchial hyperreactivity (BHR) or bronchial hyperresponsiveness.

You can minimize your wheezing in cold weather by keeping good control of your asthma with regular treatment, and if necessary by taking extra reliever treatment before you go out into cold air (see Chapter 2 for more about relievers).

Can 'living flame' gas fires make my asthma worse?

We are not aware of any published information on this topic. As we state many times in this book, people vary so much that some trigger factors may be rare in the general population, but very important to individuals.

It seems likely that a 'living flame' gas fire is no different from any other gas fire in terms of pollution or fumes. Any gas fire is more likely to cause a problem if it is old or has not been properly serviced. If this is not the case for your gas fire, it seems to us that a possible explanation for your asthma becoming worse when it is on is the fact that air temperature and humidity in the room will alter appreciably. Changes in air temperature and humidity are quite potent triggers for asthma symptoms.

I always get attacks in winter. Why is this?

There are several possible reasons but there are three main ones:

- Your attacks probably result from a cold which goes on to your chest. An upper respiratory tract infection (common cold) is responsible, and is the most common asthma trigger. In the winter months there are more of these viral infections around than at any other time of year.
- Cold air is an important trigger factor and, of course, this will affect your chest more in the winter than at other times of the year.
- Finally, house dust mite numbers are at their highest in the early part of the winter, when the heating is switched on.

I am 42 years old, and have a part time job. Why does being overtired cause me to have an asthma attack?

Being overtired in itself should not cause you to have an asthma attack, but there are reasons why this might seem to be the case. Asthma can be triggered by many different factors and it is possible that when you are overtired, stress or other emotional upsets may play an important role. Equally it might be that you feel very tired after you have exercised or that you feel 'run down' while suffering from an upper respiratory tract infection (common cold, or similar virus infection). Both exercise and virus infections are well known asthma triggers.

People with asthma sometimes don't realize that their asthma is getting worse, because it happens gradually over a period of time.

They may adjust and cope with their symptoms until the asthma becomes quite bad. If you are one of these people, it is more likely to be that the worsening asthma is causing your tiredness, rather than that overtiredness is causing your asthma.

Why, when my asthma is caused by allergies, do I have attacks when I get excited or upset?

Just because your asthma is mainly triggered by allergies, it does not mean that other trigger factors cannot cause symptoms, or even attacks. Most commonly, people with allergic asthma find that colds or other virus infections make their asthma worse. However, around 40% of people with asthma report that emotional stress or overexcitement can make their asthma worse. These are more likely to affect you if your asthma is unstable and poorly controlled. On the other hand, if your asthma is well controlled, you are less likely to get stress-related symptoms.

Why do some things (e.g. cat hairs) trigger off my asthma symptoms, yet similar things (e.g. dog hairs) do not?

We do not know the complete answer here. There is so much variation between individuals, and also in individual cases at different times, that it becomes impossible to cover all the factors involved.

Not everyone is allergic to the same substances and just what triggers off your asthma will depend on your particular allergy. Most domestic pets with hair or feathers can be a source of problems because they live in such close proximity to people. Interestingly, male animals appear to cause more allergic asthma than females!

Cats are the most common trigger of animal allergy, particularly in children. Many people are allergic only to kittens, or to certain breeds, particularly Siamese and Burmese. Dogs (particularly the short haired varieties), horses, hamsters and guinea pigs can also cause allergic asthma.

Although hair, skin and scurf generate the allergy in most cases, surprisingly it has been shown for cats that the allergen is in the saliva. When the animal washes itself, the allergen becomes stuck on to the fur, and from there it comes more easily into contact with the person with asthma.

Is it really asthma, and is there more than one type?

How do doctors diagnose asthma?

There is more than one way of diagnosing asthma. The medical history is often enough in itself to enable the diagnosis to be made. There are many clues in the past medical history to suggest asthma as the cause of someone's problem.

Asthma is a chronic (long lasting) condition, in which sufferers may be free from symptoms for periods of time and very ill at others. They will usually have a pattern of symptoms which come and go.

In asthma the symptoms often get worse with exercise, laughter, colds, or in a smoky or dusty room. Anyone who suffers lots of coughs, or who gets wheezy repeatedly should be suspected of having asthma until proved otherwise.

The diagnosis can be confirmed in two ways. One way is to see if anti-asthma medication clears the symptoms. Sometimes this may need to be taken for weeks before it starts to work. In young children this is the most suitable way of making the diagnosis.

A more convincing way in older children and adults is by the use of peak flow meter readings. The peak expiratory flow is a measurement of how narrowed the airways in the lungs are. If the airways are narrowed, as in episodes of asthma, then the readings are lower. In asthma, peak flow readings vary between good times and bad times by more than 15%. If this can be demonstrated, then the condition is diagnosed. This may occur during the consultation with the doctor, but more often someone will be asked to keep a 'peak flow diary'.

There are three important changes on a peak flow diary for doctors to look out for in the diagnosis of asthma:

1 a variation between readings of more than 15%;
2 increased difference between the morning and evening readings;
3 early *morning dips* in the readings.

For example in the peak flow chart in Figure 1.4 the highest reading is 400 and the lowest is 300:

$$\frac{\text{Highest} - \text{lowest}}{\text{Highest}} \times 100 = \frac{400 - 300}{400} \times 100 = 25\% \text{ variation}$$

The variation between highest and lowest readings is much greater than 15%, confirming the diagnosis of asthma.

The peak flow chart can also be used to confirm that someone has asthma by following their response to anti-asthma treatment.

1 It confirms the diagnosis if anti-asthma medication makes you better. Sometimes this medication needs to be continued for quite a few weeks, or even months, before it starts to work.
2 If the peak expiratory flow improves with treatment then the diagnosis is confirmed. Three things to watch for improvement on a peak flow chart are an increase in the readings (this should be at least 15% for the diagnosis to be confirmed); a decreased

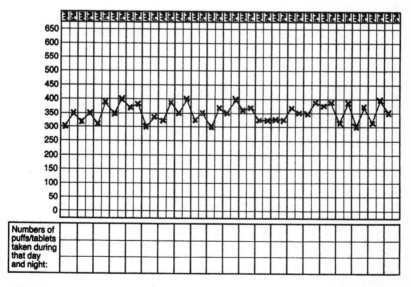

Figure 1.4 This chart shows peak flow readings which are between 400 and 300 litres per minute. They vary by more than 15%, confirming that the diagnosis is asthma.

gap between the morning and evening readings; and a great reduction in early morning dips in the readings (see Figure 3.7).

Figure 1.5 shows two of these things (see also Figures 3.6, 3.9, 3.10 and 6.1). This man saw his doctor on the sixth of the month. The doctor confirmed the diagnosis of asthma from the medical history and started treatment with an inhaled steroid at two puffs twice a day. The man was asked to keep a record of his morning and evening peak flows. The graph shows the improvement in readings, which gradually increase from 300 to around 500. The gap between the morning and evening readings gets less during the following weeks and the readings level off after about four weeks.

Have I really got asthma?

A lot of people ask this question, especially if they have only mild

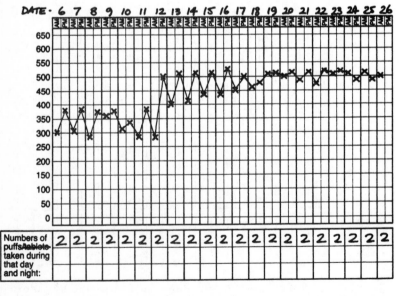

Figure 1.5   Peak flow chart showing gradual improvement in readings after starting asthma treatment. This confirms the diagnosis of asthma.

or occasional symptoms. They may believe that to have asthma you need to be severely ill and incapacitated, but they are wrong. Most people with asthma have mild asthma most of the time.

There are certain pointers which will establish whether or not you really do have asthma. The story you tell the doctor about the nature and frequency of your symptoms and what brings them on should alert him or her to the diagnosis. You may well be asked to blow into a peak flow meter for a week or so, and to record your measurements twice a day. Your doctor will be looking to see how much your readings vary between the morning and the evening, and from day to day. If they vary by 15% or more asthma is by far the most likely cause.

Another way of confirming that you really do have asthma is for your doctor to measure your peak flow before and after exercise or treatment (exercise testing or reversibility testing). We need to be careful with interpreting these tests, because although a positive result confirms asthma, if they are not conclusive they do not necessarily rule it out.

Do different people have different asthma, or is it all the same?

This question is in two parts, and really there are two ways of answering it. In one sense, all people with asthma have the same condition. They have that combination of twitchy airways and overproduction of mucus from swollen airway linings which leads to the symptoms of asthma. However, there is an enormous range of asthma amongst different people. The speed with which the condition develops, the triggers that continue to provoke it, and the responses to different treatments all vary widely between individuals.

Asthma can be categorized in different ways: extrinsic (allergic) versus intrinsic (non-allergic) according to what usually triggers episodes; mild, moderate or severe, according to the seriousness of the episodes; easy, difficult or brittle, according to the way it responds to treatments.

One form of asthma which is sometimes regarded as a different condition is *occupational asthma*, because it is more clearly defined in terms of its cause. This is asthma that starts as a result of something in the workplace, which people do not come up against anywhere else. A good example of occupational asthma is that caused by fumes from soldering work in electrical companies. Occupational asthma may disappear completely if the affected person is no longer exposed to the cause.

I have heard people talking about extrinsic and intrinsic asthma. What do they mean?

We do tend to categorize asthma into one of two groups, called extrinsic and intrinsic. The problem with doing this is that there is often overlap between the two.

The most obvious feature about extrinsic asthma is that it is triggered by external or 'outside' factors to specific allergens such as pollen and house dust mite. It tends to start in childhood and often occurs along with eczema and hay fever. If skin tests for allergy are carried out they are positive to one or more of the common allergens. Symptoms of extrinsic asthma tend to come and go and sometimes the affected person is completely free of them.

Intrinsic asthma tends to start later in life and skin tests, if they are carried out, are usually negative. Unfortunately for the sufferer the symptoms are usually persistent and there may be no easily identifiable triggers, except for common colds. Interestingly, people with this type of asthma are sometimes sensitive to aspirin, and some develop little non-malignant (non-cancerous) growths in the nose called nasal polyps.

Because there may be such an overlap between the groups, with asthma sufferers showing features of both, many doctors regard this division into two types as unhelpful.

What is the most common cause of asthma?

We need to distinguish between the **cause** of asthma, and the trigger factors for symptoms and attacks.

Some people are born with a tendency to develop asthma later in life. Usually this comes out in childhood, but in some cases it does not become obvious until they are much older. If a person has inherited this tendency, then something else is needed to set off the asthma – to uncover it from its 'tendency' into a real life condition. If we think of this event as the 'cause' of asthma, then without doubt, the most common cause is a virus infection. This sounds very dull! Doctors seem to spend most of their time telling patients that problems are caused by viruses – and yet in the case of asthma it is probably true. Certain virus infections of the nose, throat and lungs seem to have the ability to uncover asthma in a person who is already prone to it. One example in children is a group of viruses called 'rhinoviruses', which are known to cause wheezing episodes in those who are vulnerable. This whole process is sometimes referred to as the 'inception' of asthma.

Trigger factors spark off episodes of asthma and are quite different (see the section on *Triggers*) and yet, of all the possible triggers, virus infections are probably the commonest! Research has shown that over 80% of uncontrolled asthma episodes in schoolchildren are linked with viruses. Similarly, many episodes of adult asthma are linked with virus infections. So viruses are extremely important in setting off asthma in the first place, and also in triggering episodes and attacks.

All three of my children have asthma, but one of them is much worse than the other two. Why is that?

We cannot really explain why one of your three children should have asthma so much worse than the other two, but it is not uncommon for this to be the case.

It may be helpful to think of asthma occurring as a result of the way our bodies react to outside stimuli (or triggers), be they allergens, viruses, pollution or anything else. No two people are the same, and so everybody with asthma is different in the way they react to triggers. Some people may be well for most of the time, but be prone to sudden severe attacks. Others have more chronic, ongoing symptoms, but are less likely to have acute severe episodes. Some people respond much better than others to the asthma treatments we have available.

There are circumstances under which people are more likely to suffer from severe asthma. If there is a strong family history, with other family members having severe asthma, the chances of severe asthma are greater. If the asthma is of many years' duration, and not well controlled, then it is more likely that the lungs will have become permanently affected, and so acute attacks will be more severe. Finally elderly people who develop asthma alongside other chronic lung conditions such as emphysema or chronic bronchitis have much less lung function in reserve, so their asthma is more likely to have severe effects.

Can you please explain the difference between the 'wheezy' and the 'quiet' types of asthma? Having experienced both, I find the latter more troublesome in later life.

This is a very important question. When your airways are slightly narrowed, they produce a wheezing or whistling sound during breathing in and out. The breathing in this type of asthma is noisy, and it is very easy to tell that you are suffering from asthma. When your asthma is severe, some airways are almost closed, and very little air can move in and out of the lungs. If this happens your breathing becomes very quiet, and it may not be so obvious that your asthma is bad. You might be having difficulty in breathing or speaking, and you may even be a blue colour around your lips and tongue. A very low peak flow reading is the best way to confirm that your asthma is indeed very bad. This can be a very dangerous condition, especially in an acute attack when you need urgent medical help.

In your own case, however, this more severe form of asthma has probably developed over some years, but it indicates that your airways are quite severely narrowed. This is why you find it more difficult to deal with than the 'wheezy' type you had when you were younger.

Inheritance

Why have I got asthma?

Many people feel singled out in suffering from asthma, while many others almost expect it because it runs so strongly in their families. Perhaps around 40% of the population in the UK have the potential to develop asthma and so no-one should feel singled out or unusual because they suffer from it. You have inherited a tendency to get asthma, and something has switched it on or triggered it. How we acquire the asthma tendency is not fully understood. We know that some of our characteristics (like the colour of our eyes) and some rare diseases (such as haemophilia) can be caused by inheriting single *genes*. Individual genes which are important in the process are being identified, but it is probably a combination of a number of different genes that determines the asthma tendency.

So first of all you need to have inherited the tendency to get asthma and then something must convert that tendency into the actual condition. The 'something' is almost as mysterious as the way in which we inherit the tendency! It seems that in children certain virus infections of the respiratory system (e.g. colds) spark off changes in the linings of the airways, and this sets off the symptoms of asthma. This may also occur in adults, but there are other factors responsible, such as allergies or working in certain occupations. Some people with the inherited tendency to develop asthma may go through their entire lives and not get asthma, despite encountering these factors many times. This is just one more of the mysteries underlining how little we really understand about the causes of asthma.

What are the chances of a baby I might have in the future developing asthma?

You have a much greater chance of having a child with asthma if you or any of your close relatives already have asthma. It is also more likely if you or your husband are atopic. Being atopic in itself does not automatically cause asthma, but it does make you more susceptible to developing conditions such as asthma, eczema and hay fever. If you and your partner are both atopic, then your baby will have about a one in two chance of developing an atopic condition – but, of course, this may or may not be asthma.

Studies carried out on the families of infants with asthma suggest there is an inherited (or genetic) element which influences the development of what is known as bronchial hyperreactivity (or 'twitchy airways'). This inherited element probably has an effect only if something in the environment influences it, in the way we have described in the previous question.

**I have been well all of my life. I have no relatives with
asthma, and now at the age of 42 I have developed asthma.
Why me?**

Asthma is very common, and probably becoming even more
common, so you might almost ask 'why not me?'.

Probably between two and three million people in this country
have asthma, around one in 20 of these are adults, and at least one
in 10 are children. Even though it is so common, this does not of
course automatically make it more acceptable to you or your
family.

The severity of asthma varies enormously. It can be mild but it
can also be very disabling, disruptive, dangerous and frightening.
Many people feel very worried and depressed when they are told
they have asthma. Others feel angry and aggressive. In addition to
this, some parents may feel guilty that they have 'passed it on' to
their child or children. These feelings are a very natural reaction.
However, once people know more about their asthma and the fact
that it can usually be treated successfully, then most of them find
that these feelings subside, and that they 'come to terms' with
their asthma.

Having asthma can still carry an unnecessary stigma and some
people feel ashamed and wish to avoid anyone knowing about it.
This is regrettable, and it could well date from the era when
asthma was considered (wrongly) to be psychological and 'nervous' asthma was thought to be the fault of the patient, not the
environment or their genes. If you have asthma, it is nobody's
fault.

It is worth remembering that the aim of modern asthma management is for you to be free from symptoms at all times and to be
able to lead a full life with no restrictions.

**As asthma runs in families is there anything I can do to
prevent my children from getting it?**

There is some evidence to suggest that children who are
exposed to allergy-causing substances in the first few months of
life are more likely to develop asthma later in childhood. This is
particularly likely in those where there is a history of allergy in
the family. Babies born between March and May are exposed to

high pollen levels and those born in the early winter months arrive when the house dust mite is at its most active. So if you want to try and reduce the chances of your child developing an allergic condition (asthma, hay fever or eczema), then you should plan the birth for between December and February – no easy task!

More reasonably, you can avoid smoking. It is known that smoking in pregnancy and during the early months of babies' lives increases allergy antibodies (substances produced by the immune system) in them. It can also be helpful to reduce exposure to some allergens (e.g. pets or house dust) during infancy. Breastfeeding your baby for at least the first three months will reduce the chances of eczema developing, but does not appear to protect against asthma.

Some crucial research studies are being carried out to determine whether it is possible to prevent the development of asthma by avoiding important allergens during pregnancy and in early infancy. The main findings so far link smoking parents (particularly mothers) with increased numbers of children with asthma. Therefore parents of young children should not smoke, particularly if they or their relatives have asthma, hay fever or allergies.

I already have one child with asthma. If I have other children in the future, is it likely that they will have it too?

Yes, it is. Asthma is more common in families where someone already has the condition. So if you have at least one relative with asthma then you have an increased chance of having a child with asthma. A family history of eczema, hay fever and other allergic conditions (e.g. to medicines like penicillin or to bee sting) increases the possibility of having a child with asthma.

There are other things which may be associated with asthma, and which may affect your children. Bottle-fed babies are more likely to develop allergic problems (and therefore asthma) than those who are breast fed for more than three months. Children in small families from more affluent homes seem more prone to allergic conditions. Children from families who smoke have more chest problems, including asthma.

I have had asthma since childhood. Will my children have asthma?

There is no doubt that all atopic (allergic) conditions such as asthma, hay fever and eczema do tend to run in families. So if both parents are atopic they have a much greater chance of having a child with asthma (or any of the other atopic conditions for that matter) than if they were non-atopic.

Recent research has shown that, of the atopic children who took part in a study in Oxford, 90% of them had at least one parent who was atopic; atopy occurred in 33% of parents with non-atopic children. Further research showed that atopy occurred in about 60% of children born to couples in which one parent was atopic and the other non-atopic.

You will find out more information about atopy in the section on *Related conditions*.

I'm over 60 and have just been diagnosed as having asthma. I've never had any problem before – why have I got asthma now?

Asthma can occur at any time of life. It may appear for the first time in a premature baby or in an octogenarian. What we can't tell you is why **you** have developed asthma **now**. One of the commonest reasons for people to develop asthma for the first time between the ages of 40 and 60 years (*late onset asthma*) is as a result of a severe episode of 'bronchitis', or a chest infection. They may seem to make a slow but full recovery, only for their chesty symptoms to return. The coughing, wheezing and breathlessness can be very distressing, with particularly marked symptoms at night. You haven't said whether you are a man or a woman, but interestingly more women than men in your age group develop asthma. Unfortunately many adults who develop asthma are wrongly diagnosed as having bronchitis, even if they have never smoked or lived and worked in a polluted environment. If bronchitis is diagnosed, this often means that the doctor doesn't prescribe anti-asthma drugs. It is good that your condition has been diagnosed definitely, because now at least you should receive the correct treatment.

All in the mind?

To what extent is my asthma psychosomatic?

If by this you mean 'Is my asthma all in my mind?' the answer is definitely no. However, certain psychological factors such as stress can trigger asthma attacks. This happens in people who already have asthma in the first place.

It is important to understand that asthma does have a strong psychological effect on sufferers and their families. Most people with asthma need to take regular medication and, if they forget, they may become very ill. Even if they do take regular treatment they may still occasionally get a severe attack. These attacks may start suddenly without warning and this can be a very stressful on the whole family. Some families have experience of terrifying attacks, spoilt holidays and lack of sleep. These things have a profound effect on their lives. Regular monitoring (see Chapter 3) and effective treatment (see Chapter 2) will minimize these problems, and so reduce the amount of stress they would otherwise cause.

Are nervous people more prone to asthma?

No. However, there are some features of asthma which lead people to associate asthma with nervous problems. Breathlessness, although due to physical causes, is sometimes seen by people who do not have asthma as a sign of nervousness.

Life with asthma can be very unpredictable. The disease can change from day to day – one day all will be well, and on another an acute asthma attack may occur. This is enough to make anyone nervous. Research has shown that severe asthma in children is associated with depression in mothers. It is not known which of these conditions comes first. Does the depressed mother make her child more liable to develop asthma, or does the fact that her child has severe asthma cause a sense of depression in the mother? Further research is needed to answer these questions.

I developed asthma at the age of 10, after the death of my mother. Could some other trauma cause it to go away?

Asthma is an unpredictable condition. There may be many reasons why it begins, and just as many for its disappearance. It does sometimes develop following a tragedy or an accident. Probably a combination of circumstances is needed for the asthma to appear at this time, but the other factors may not be so obvious. It may have seemed as if the loss of your mother was the only factor, but there may have been others. Sadly, it is less likely that further trauma will cause it to go away.

I have asthma and when my children were born I had post-natal depression. I have heard that asthma is a nervous condition, so is there a link?

We do not believe that asthma is a nervous condition. However, it is accepted that depression can make some people's asthma worse. It is important to realize, however, that depression on its own will not cause asthma in someone who has never had it before. Both conditions are very common. Asthma occurs in approximately 5% of the adult population, and postnatal depression affects around 10% of women in the year after childbirth. So it is not surprising that the two conditions occur together in some cases. However, there is no important link between asthma and postnatal depression, and mothers with and without asthma have the same risk of developing it.

Is stress in my marriage responsible for the poor control of my asthma?

There is no doubt that, in some people, stress and other psychological factors can make asthma worse and can lead to constant symptoms. For most people, most of the time, emotional stresses have little or no effect on their asthma. Usually there are several trigger factors working at the same time, and emotional upset may be just be one of them. The stress in your marriage may be contributing to the poor control of your asthma, but we doubt whether it is the sole cause. In any case it will be a good idea to see your doctor to get your asthma under better control, rather than just putting up with it. It will make one less problem for you to deal with.

Is it usual for people with asthma also to suffer from claustrophobia, as I do?

Not really! Asthma is such a common problem that many people have other conditions which are in no way linked to their asthma. Claustrophobia is a very unpleasant, occasionally serious condition which is also common, though not as common as asthma. It involves a fear of closed or confined spaces which is extreme (as far as people who **don't** have claustrophobia are concerned!). Inevitably some people will suffer from both conditions, but not many. We wonder if you are suffering from feelings of suffocation during attacks, rather than true claustrophobia. This is much more common. Many people feel like this during attacks, and feel the understandable urge to find open space and fresh air.

Related conditions

Are there any ailments or illnesses associated with asthma?

Yes – there are three common and very important conditions that are closely associated with asthma. These are eczema, hay fever and general allergy to various substances (for example cats, dogs, horses, house dust mite and some medicines).

Another very important condition that may be difficult to separate from asthma is chronic bronchitis. The two conditions often occur together, particularly in the elderly.

There are other conditions which are less common, but also related to asthma, including polyps (small non-cancerous growths) in the nose and allergic skin conditions such as urticaria. Urticaria consists of raised blotchy patches on the skin looking very much like nettle rash.

Other important chronic conditions, such as high blood pressure and diabetes, are not directly related, but because (like asthma) they are common, they frequently occur in those with asthma.

How do I know it's asthma and not allergy?

Allergy occurs when the body reacts against an external substance. This might be pollen, dust or medicines, e.g. penicillin. The allergic reaction may take the form of a runny nose, a skin rash, swelling eyelids or wheezing. The allergic reaction may start an asthma attack or an episode of uncontrolled asthma. Allergy is one of the triggers of asthma and therefore may occur at the same time. The best way to tell if it is asthma is to use a peak flow chart, using the best of three readings in the morning and the evening (or more frequently if symptoms are bad). In asthma the peak flow goes up and down – it does not remain steady. A variation of 15% or more shows that the asthma is out of control and causing the symptoms. You will find more details in the section on *Peak flow monitoring* in Chapter 3.

What is atopy?

Atopy is not a disease; it refers to an inherited tendency (or pre-disposition), that makes people more likely to develop an allergic disorder. It does not follow that, if you are found to be atopic, you will have one of the allergic diseases such as asthma, hay fever or eczema. People who are atopic have the ability to produce the allergy antibody called immunoglobulin E, or IgE.

Genetic research suggests that the tendency to develop asthma is inherited separately from the atopic tendency. However, if you have both, it is much more likely that you will develop asthma. That's why it is common for the three conditions of asthma, hay fever and eczema to exist together. Not all atopic people have asthma and not all people with asthma are atopic (although around 75% are). It has also been suggested that if you get a cold (virus infection) at a time when you are exposed to an allergen (like pollen), you are more likely to develop asthma.

Highly atopic people often have parents with atopic disease and it is very likely that they will develop asthma, and will continue to have it together with other allergic disorders for the rest of their life.

One way to tell whether a person is atopic or not is a test in which the skin is pricked through solutions of allergen dropped onto the skin. This is called *skin prick testing* and is carried out either in general practice or, more usually, in hospital. In atopic people, skin prick tests will nearly always give a positive result (a raised weal like a nettle sting).

What is the connection between asthma and eczema? Is asthma a kind of internal eczema?

A large proportion of the population, perhaps up to 30%, are 'atopic', as described in the previous question. To be atopic is to have inherited a tendency to develop an allergic illness. The most common of these illnesses are eczema and hay fever. Asthma is an inherited condition which is very often associated with atopy. It is thought that asthma is more liable to appear if the person is also atopic. In other words, having one condition, atopy, makes the development of the other, asthma, more likely. Atopic eczema occurs particularly in children, and is very common. Inevitably, many children have both asthma and eczema. Your suggestion that asthma is a kind of internal eczema is a very good one. Eczema causes red, irritable, itchy, inflamed skin. This is very much like the inflammation that occurs in the linings of the airways in asthma. So the two conditions are connected, and in many ways they are similar.

How does asthma differ from other chest conditions and breathing difficulties?

Asthma is a condition in which symptoms are caused by narrowing of the airways which is **reversible**. This means that symptoms come and go, and for much of the time people with asthma are completely well. For example, athletes with asthma are able to perform at their peak when their asthma is well controlled. This is the main difference between asthma and other chest conditions.

Chronic bronchitis is another condition affecting the airways, but it is not reversible. Chronic bronchitis and emphysema (which is discussed in the next question) are both conditions which usually affect older adults, often those who have smoked for many years. These diseases are permanent and treatment can only be used to lessen symptoms. They tend to be more severe than asthma, and less responsive to treatment.

Cystic fibrosis is an inherited condition where there is a problem with the proteins made by the body. The result is that mucus is very sticky, and blocks up the air passages. Children with cystic fibrosis may first come to the doctor with symptoms similar to asthma, although usually they are more unwell. Doctors will be aware of this condition and will arrange for tests to be done in any children suspected of having cystic fibrosis.

Air pollution causes a lot of chest symptoms. Miners and other industrial workers exposed to lots of fumes and dust also suffer from problems with their chests, often developing scar tissue in the lungs as well as emphysema. *Passive smoking* is responsible for a lot of chest illness. Both air pollution and passive smoking worsen asthma.

Heart disease may cause difficulty in breathing. This usually results from the collection of fluid in the lungs when the heart is not pumping effectively. One form of this, acute heart failure, used to be known as 'cardiac asthma', but it is a completely different condition, and the term is hardly ever used these days.

I have emphysema. What is it, and is it associated with asthma?

Smoking is the main cause of emphysema. It is congenital in some people (i.e. some people are born with a tendency to develop it) and caused by air pollution or certain occupations (like mining) in others. In emphysema the walls of the air spaces in the lungs are damaged. These air spaces, called alveoli, are normally very elastic. The lungs inflate when air is breathed in and contract when air is expelled. This elasticity is destroyed in emphysema and the lungs become very large due to overexpansion. The damaged areas of the lungs cannot trans-port oxygen into, and waste products out of, the blood, so peo-ple with emphysema become short of oxygen, their bodies cannot function normally, and they are often very tired and lethargic.

The relationship between emphysema and asthma is unclear. There is some evidence which suggests that asthma can, when severe and persistent, cause scar tissue to form in the lungs. This scar tissue can damage the walls of the air spaces and passages and this may lead to emphysema. It is not known for sure why this scar tissue develops in asthma, but it is believed to be a result of the inflammation which occurs. Most asthma experts now advise that treatments to reduce inflammation should be used regularly to try to avoid scar tissue developing.

I'm 65. How do I know its asthma and not emphysema?

It can be difficult to tell the difference between Chronic Obstructive Pulmonary Disease (i.e. COPD; emphysema is one of the causes of COPD) and asthma. Both conditions cause airway obstruction. COPD is more common in older people. People with COPD have usually smoked in the past (or are current smokers). In asthma the obstruction is reversible, whilst in emphysema (or COPD) this is fixed. Asthma can usually be diagnosed on the medical history and peak expiratory flow tests; spirometry (special breathing tests using equipment called a spirometer) is used for diagnosing COPD. Symptoms in both conditions usually improve with reliever drugs (like salbutamol and terbutaline). Asthma usually improves with inhaled anti-inflammatory treatment (like inhaled topical steroids), while emphysema sometimes does.

It is important to get the diagnosis right because it is inappropriate to take long-term treatment for asthma if you have COPD. Some people with COPD do improve with anti-asthma treatment, and therefore the doctor would often encourage a patient to try this treatment for a while (a trial of therapy). This sometimes includes a short course of cortisone tablets. If your lung function does improve while you are taking this treatment, it is well worthwhile continuing on some form of anti-inflammatory treatment. The opposite is not true. If the medication has not proved to be of benefit, there is little advantage to be gained by continuing, at the risk of getting unwanted side effects. Episodes of asthma and COPD are treated differently. Asthma treatment is dealt with in this book; COPD episodes are treated mainly with high doses of reliever drugs, oxygen, and sometimes with steroids and antibiotics. Antibiotics are not very often useful in asthma attacks or flare-ups.

In elderly people, is there a link between having asthma now, and having had TB in the past?

The only possible link is an indirect one. Tuberculosis (TB) infection can be brought on by steroid tablets used to treat asthma in older patients. It is rare, and can only happen if the person concerned has suffered from TB in the past.

Before immunisation and modern drugs were available, TB used to be very common, and a major cause of early death. The first contact with TB (called primary TB) usually occurred in childhood, and nearly always left a small scar in the lungs. This scar could provide the beginnings of more serious TB infection later in life. Quite a number of elderly people have the scar of healed primary TB in their lungs (this is rare in middle aged and young people). This scar hardly ever gives rise to any symptoms or problems. However, one known trigger for 'awakening' old TB is treatment with steroids. These, of course, are used often in the treatment of severe episodes of asthma.

Anyone who has had TB in the past should tell their doctor about this, particularly if they also have asthma. It may be necessary to have a chest X-ray regularly if steroid tablets are required for asthma. TB is a very serious infection, but it can now be cured completely by tablets, as long as it is recognized.

There is no direct link between TB and asthma. In other words, if you have asthma, you are no more likely than anyone else of your own age to get TB.

Some figures about asthma

How many people have asthma?

This depends very much on how you define asthma. About one third of the population in the UK have wheezing at some stage of their lives. Do they all have asthma? Probably not!

Asthma comes and goes during someone's lifetime. Many children who have asthma go into a quiet stage (into remission) as they approach puberty. The problem therefore is to decide where to draw the line in answering the question. Do we look at just those people who have asthma at any one time or at all those who have ever had asthma?

Between one in seven UK children have asthma (about 1.5 million children). Yet about one in three children have wheezed at some time in their lives. About one in 25 adults (over 16 years), i.e. over 1.9 million adults in the UK, are affected by asthma.

Using these figures, we can calculate that in the UK there are between two and three million people with asthma at the present time.

Is asthma a killer?

Yes, asthma can result in death. It is the cause of around 1600 deaths each year in the UK. The majority of these deaths occur in the elderly but around one in three occur in people aged under 65, and most of these are believed to be preventable.

Of course, death during an acute asthma attack is a devastating tragedy. We must bear in mind that, in view of the numbers of people affected by asthma, fatal attacks are **very rare**. The younger the age group studied, the fewer the deaths that occur; so that in youngsters and children there are only around 30 deaths per year.

Nevertheless, it is important to be aware that asthma can be a life-threatening condition. Studies have shown that many people dying from asthma failed to recognize danger signals, and did not increase their use of medication as they should have done. Many did not call for medical help early enough, and unfortunately relatives, ambulance staff and doctors often failed to appreciate the urgency of the problem.

It is vital, therefore, that if you have asthma, you and your friends and relatives should learn as much about the condition as possible. You – and they – should know how to recognize when asthma is going out of control and, ideally, know what to do if this happens. Failing this, they must always ask for medical advice as soon as possible. Death from asthma is a rare event but it can, and does, happen.

Is asthma more severe these days?

This is a difficult question to answer because there are no clear ways of measuring severity of asthma. There is certainly more asthma around nowadays and there are lots of explanations for this. Air pollution causes more people to suffer from their asthma. There is no evidence to prove that air pollution causes asthma.

About the only way we can gauge the severity of asthma is by its effect upon people's lives (deaths, hospital admissions and emergencies, and symptoms).

Asthma deaths occur as frequently as they did 25 years ago. In the UK there is one death from asthma every six hours.

There are more hospital admissions for asthma in the UK than in the past. This may be due to increased severity of asthma but there are a few other possible explanations. It may also be due to increased awareness of the dangers of undertreatment of asthma, and so people with asthma and health professionals may be less reluctant to use the hospital services than before.

Surveys show that most people with asthma have symptoms from asthma every day of their lives. These people limit their physical activities because of these symptoms; they miss schooling and are frequently absent from work as a result. In nearly all cases this should be unnecessary. Effective management of asthma may remove all of these problems.

Is asthma more common in some parts of the country than others?

It is not possible to answer this question with any certainty. Research is under way to try to find out, and before too long we may know for sure. We do know that there are differences across the country in the way that asthma is diagnosed and treated. Some regions have much higher hospital admission rates than others, but this cannot be taken as an indication that asthma is more common or more severe in these regions.

In children a number of surveys has been carried out, and it seems the prevalence of asthma is broadly similar, at about 10–15% in areas of the UK as far apart as London, the East Midlands, the North East, Wales and Scotland.

Do some countries have more sufferers and, if so, why?

There are wide variations around the world in the proportions of populations suffering from asthma. In some countries such as New Zealand and Australia the proportions are high (17% and 13% respectively). At one time, some 45% of the inhabitants of the South Atlantic island of Tristan da Cunha were affected by asthma, as a result of much interbreeding in the small population. In India, Scandinavian countries and rural African countries the proportions are low (under 3%). In other countries, such as the UK, over 7% of the population suffer from asthma. The proportion of a population suffering from a condition is referred to as the *prevalence* so we say that the prevalence of asthma in the UK is around 6–7%.

That much is clear, but we cannot really explain why these variations occur. Some, but not all, of the variation has to do with climate, urbanization and the 'genetic stock' of the population. Asthma is, to a large extent, an inherited condition. In those countries where few people have the genes giving the tendency to get asthma, few children will inherit those genes. The different use of the term asthma is another reason for the wide variations found across the world. It may seem remarkable, but international conferences of experts have found it difficult to agree on an exact definition of asthma. Different countries and different studies have used many descriptions. This makes it very hard to judge the variations between countries. Another reason is that the severity of asthma seems to vary from country to country. For example in New Zealand, people seem to suffer from a more severe form of asthma than in other parts of the world.

Does asthma go in seven year cycles – or is this a myth?

We have come across this one before, but we believe it is a myth! Asthma does tend to go into remission (stops causing symptoms) for periods of time, particularly in older children as they reach puberty. This remission may last for months or for many years, but we know of no evidence to suggest that it tends to last for seven years. It is no more likely than seven years' bad luck from a broken mirror!

2
Treatment

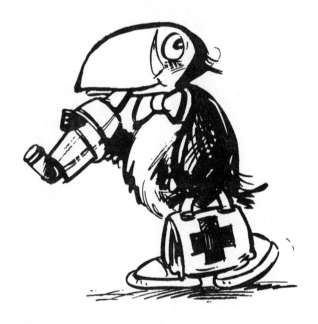

Introduction

This chapter deals with the main medical treatments for asthma available in the UK. Non-drug treatments and complementary therapies are covered in more detail in Chapter 7.

There are dozens of drugs available to treat asthma in the UK but in practice there are only a few that are really in common use. If your own treatment is not named in the book it does not mean that you are receiving an unacceptable drug, just that for reasons of space we are unable to include all possible drugs in the answer to each question. An added complication is that each drug has a minimum of two names! The *generic name* is the basic drug name, but each drug also has a *brand name*, given by the manufacturer (Plate 1). For example, the most frequently prescribed drug for asthma is salbutamol (generic name). This is best known by the brand name Ventolin, used by its leading manufacturer, but also has the name Aerolin when marketed by a different company. We have decided against using only generic names, because most people are familiar with brand names – indeed most of the questions we have received on treatment have used brand names. The most frequently prescribed drugs for asthma in the UK are: Ventolin Evohaler, Salamol (generic name salbutamol); Bricanyl (terbutaline); Becotide, Beclazone, Becloforte, Qvar (beclomethasone); Flixotide (fluticasone propionate); Pulmicort (budesonide); Intal (sodium cromoglycate); Serevent (salmeterol); Foradil (eformoterol fumarate); and Tilade (nedocromil). The tablets Singulair (montelukast) and (Zafirlukast) are being prescribed with increasing frequency. There are many other important drugs, and there are questions about them in this chapter.

At present, inhaled asthma drugs are placed into one of two categories – preventers and relievers.

Preventer drugs are taken by the inhaled route. They are either *steroids* (such as Aerobec, Becotide, Filair, Flixotide and Pulmicort) or belong to another *anti-inflammatory* group (Intal or Tilade). They must be taken regularly to have their maximum effect in preventing symptoms.

Reliever drugs are there to relieve symptoms when they occur, and therefore do not need to be taken regularly. In fact, some evidence suggests that they are more effective when they are taken occasionally rather than regularly.

Some reliever drugs are long acting. Serevent (salmeterol), Oxis and Foradil (eformoterol fumarate) are three examples of these drugs. They are similar in action to the relievers, but are longer acting (they work for 12 hous compared to 4 hours for most relievers). *Long acting relievers* are normally reserved for people already taking preventers and needing extra medication. Serevent is currently available as a combination together with Flixotide;

this is called Seretide, and is usually prescribed for convenience for people already using the two drugs.

We received many questions about drug side effects. We have endeavoured to give full answers placed in the right perspective. No drug is entirely free of side effects, and we feel that we are probably more likely to have had questions from those people unlucky enough to get them, rather than the majority who do not. Our message is that the main anti-asthma drugs used today are safe and largely free from side effects. Troublesome side effects are confined to a very few people, usually those who require higher dosages because of the severity of their condition.

Drug treatments

Do I have to use my preventer inhaler all the time, even when I am well?

This is an important question, and one that is frequently asked. After all it may be hard to accept that you should take treatment all the time if you have no symptoms. Firstly, we need to remember that the aim of modern asthma management is for you to be free from symptoms at all times, and to be able to lead a full life with no restrictions. Your preventer inhaler has been pre-scribed with that purpose in mind. It works by damping down, and removing, swelling and mucus in your airways. This controls your asthma, and keeps symptoms to a minimum – **as long as it is taken regularly**. Even in mild asthma, inflammation is present in the airways of the lungs, and if left untreated could cause long-term damage. If you stop taking the preventive treatment as soon as you are well, the symptoms are likely to return. If you have been free of symptoms for months, you may well be able to reduce the treatment gradually or stop it, but this should be done in con-junction with your doctor or asthma nurse.

How often do I need to take my inhaler?

You should use your reliever inhalers, Ventolin Evohaler (generic name salbutamol) and Bricanyl (generic name terbutaline sulphate), whenever necessary. This means when you have symptoms such as cough, wheeze or shortness of breath. These drugs are very important in treating asthma attacks and can be life saving. In very severe attacks they may be used in high doses, that is 15 to 30 puffs. These reliever drugs should work quickly, and their effect should last for at least four hours. **If you need to use them more often than every four hours, then you need urgent medical help.**

Your preventer drugs must be taken regularly, even if you have no symptoms. There are two groups of preventer drugs.

- The *inhaled topical steroids*, Aerobec, Becotide, Becloforte and Filair (beclomethasone dipropionate), Flixotide (fluticasone propionate) and Pulmicort (budesonide) work for about 12 hours so they should be taken twice a day.
- Intal (sodium cromoglycate) is taken three to four times a day and before exercise. Tilade (nedocromil sodium) is used two to four times a day.

What is the difference between Becotide and Ventolin?

Becotide, Becloforte, Aerobec and Filair (beclomethasone dipropionate), Flixotide (fluticasone propionate), and Pulmicort (budesonide) are inhaled topical steroids. They are anti-inflammatory drugs which help to prevent asthma attacks. They should be used regularly, twice a day, even if there are no symptoms. They are **preventers**. The dose should be increased according to an agreed self-management plan if symptoms are worsening or more relief medication than usual is needed.

Ventolin (salbutamol) and Bricanyl (terbutaline sulphate) open up the tightened airways and are used only when symptoms happen. They are **relievers**. They should work quickly and you should feel better within 15 minutes. Their effect should last for at least four hours. These facts are important and can help you recognize when an attack is going to happen.

IF YOUR RELIEVER DRUG DOES NOT WORK QUICKLY, OR ITS EFFECTS LAST FOR LESS THAN FOUR HOURS, YOUR ASTHMA

IS UNCONTROLLED AND MEDICAL HELP IS NEEDED. TAKE EXTRA RELIEVER WHILE WAITING FOR HELP.

I only cough at night, so why do I need my preventer inhaler during the day?

Your asthma is a condition that is present most of the time, even if it is not causing you any symptoms. There is a continuing inflammation in the lining of your lungs, something like a slow burning fire where the embers are smouldering constantly and burst into flames from time to time. This inflammation causes the walls of your airways to swell up and causes phlegm (consisting of cells and mucus) to collect on them. It can vary at different times, from being very mild to severe. When your asthma is mild, then symptoms such as cough may occur only on some days or nights. When the inflammation flares up and becomes more severe, your symptoms will be present most of the day and night. The process of asthma is there in the background for most of the time, and if you get symptoms – even though it may only be at night – it is best to take regular preventive treatment.

Ventolin works better for me than Becotide so why should I take Becotide?

Ventolin and Becotide work in different ways. Ventolin is a *bronchodilator* which means that it 'dilates' or opens up the airways (a 'reliever'). Because of this it relieves asthma symptoms quickly. This is why you may feel, understandably, that this must be the best treatment. Becotide is an inhaled steroid and is purely a preventive treatment (a 'preventer'). It doesn't have an immediate effect on symptoms and needs to be taken twice daily for about a week before it begins to prevent asthma symptoms from occurring.

We do not know exactly how inhaled steroids work, but we do know that taken on a long term basis they are highly effective. In some way they control the underlying inflammation of the airways.

Most people notice that once they take inhaled steroids regularly, their asthma symptoms get better, and they have less need to use their 'reliever' inhaler. A word of caution though. It is

important to continue to use the inhaled steroid regularly. It is not
a cure, and forgetting to use your Becotide is how your asthma
begins to get out of control again.

Is it safe to use more than the stated dose of Ventolin?

It won't hurt you, but the important thing is to know why you need
to take more than the stated dose. Ventolin relieves symptoms in
most situations, particularly mild asthma. It works quickly, and is
usually very effective. However, if your asthma is becoming more
severe, you will find that Ventolin becomes less effective. It may
be tempting to keep on taking puffs of Ventolin (even though it
doesn't seem to be doing much good) but this can be dangerous,
wasting valuable time. If Ventolin is losing its effect, you should
get medical help, either from your GP or from the hospital. Once
your airways have become very narrowed by inflammation,
causing swollen tubes and excess phlegm, Ventolin (or any of the
other relievers) has very little effect. Other drugs then are needed
to treat your asthma.

The aim these days is to prevent symptoms from occurring,
thereby reducing the need to take extra Ventolin.

If I forget to take my preventer inhaler one day, should I take twice the amount the next?

Firstly let us say that we realize it is extremely easy to forget to
take your preventer inhaler – particularly when you are well,
and free from symptoms. It is of course much better if you can
remember. However, if you forget a dose of Intal or Tilade then
no benefit will be gained if you take twice the amount the next
day.

If, on the other hand, it is Becotide, Becloforte, Flixotide or
Pulmicort that you have forgotten, it may be worthwhile doubling
up the dose next time, particularly if you have developed asthma
symptoms.

What does 'when necessary' mean for my Ventolin?

'When necessary' means when you have symptoms, such as
cough, wheeze or shortness of breath.

Ventolin and Bricanyl are the two reliever drugs used most frequently in the UK. Your Ventolin can be used intermittently, only when you get symptoms, rather than regularly. Many doctors believe that it is more effective when it is used in this way.

However, if your asthma is severe or chronic, your doctor may suggest that the Ventolin should be taken regularly, with extra doses if necessary.

What should I use first – reliever or preventer inhaler?

Until fairly recently, the standard advice would have been 'always use your reliever before your preventer', because the reliever should open up the airways enough to let the preventer get deeper into your lungs. Currently though, many people do not take their reliever on a regular basis, but only if they have symptoms (or before exercise to stop symptoms developing). If your asthma is well controlled, and you have no symptoms, then the airways are fully open, and it really isn't necessary to take your reliever. Just take the preventer on its own!

I try to avoid taking my Ventolin if I feel I have been using it frequently. Does this do me more harm than actually taking it?

Yes, it does really. It is not wise to ignore symptoms of asthma. If you need extra Ventolin (or any other reliever) you or your family should recognize that your asthma is out of control. Extra medication is needed including extra preventers. It is much better for you to take it than to attempt to ignore the problem. Depending on your treatment, and your arrangements with your doctor or asthma nurse, you should either adjust your treatments in the way previously agreed, or make contact with them for further advice.

What is the difference between Beconase and Becotide?

There are a number of inhaled steroid preventers that can be used for the nose (allergic rhinitis or hayfever) as well as the chest (asthma). Beconase, Flixonase and Rhinocort are preparations for the nose whilst Becotide, Flixotide and Pulmicort are preparations for the airways of the lungs. Both types contain inhaled topical steroids, which are preventer drugs.

Becotide is used to treat asthma and Beconase is given for *rhinitis*, which is a similar condition to asthma affecting the linings of the nose. Frequently rhinitis, like asthma, is triggered by allergy. It may occur all the year round. Hay fever is the most common type, and its medical name is seasonal rhinitis.

Rhinitis can spark off an asthma attack, so it is very important to take your treatment regularly if rhinitis flares up. In seasonal rhinitis (hay fever), it is really best to start the medication just before you anticipate your symptoms, for example when the pollen counts are reported to be rising early in summer.

Becotide can be given as an aerosol spray, in *dry powder* (as in a Diskhaler – Figure 2.1 – or Rotahaler – Figure 2.2) or in a mist in a nebulizer.

Becotide, Beconase, Flixotide, Flixonase, Rhinocort and budesonide need to be taken regularly – usually twice daily (Flixonase is once daily).

Many people with asthma will find themselves using both Becotide and Beconase. This will be either because they have allergic rhinitis as well as asthma or, less commonly, because they have polyps in the nose. Polyps are large swellings of the nose. They are not cancerous. They do shrink and respond very well to steroid treatment.

If Becotide keeps my asthma under control, can it work on its own without Ventolin?

Yes it can, and increasingly we are suggesting that this is the way in which treatment should be taken – using Becotide (or another preventer) regularly, and reserving reliever treatments for when symptoms do occur. In fact it is a test of how well controlled your asthma is to ask how often you have needed to use your Ventolin. If your asthma is well controlled (and you can tell this by charting your peak flow and noting your symptoms – see Chapter 3), Becotide can maintain very good control without the necessity of using Ventolin.

However, you must remember that, however well controlled your asthma seems to be, it is a very variable condition and can

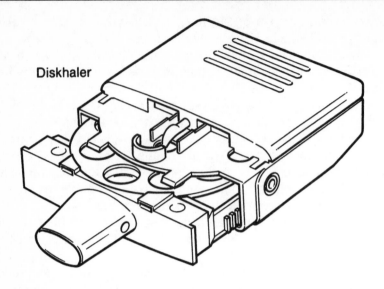

Diskhaler

Figure 2.1　How to use the Diskhaler

To load

1　Remove the mouthpiece cover, then remove the white tray by pulling it out gently and then squeezing the white ridges either side until it slides out.
2　Put the foil disk – numbers uppermost – on the wheel and slide the tray back.
3　Holding the corners of the tray, slide the tray in and out to rotate the disk until the highest number shows in the window.

To use

1　Keeping the Diskhaler level, lift the rear of the lid up as far as it will go. This will pierce the top and bottom of the blister. Close the lid.
2　Holding the Diskhaler level, breathe out gently and put the mouthpiece in your mouth. Breathe in as deeply as possible. (Do not cover the small air holes on either side of the mouthpiece.)
3　Remove the Diskhaler from your mouth and hold your breath for about 10 seconds. Slide the tray in and out ready for the next dose.

Always discuss the use of your device with your doctor or asthma nurse.

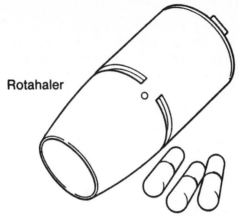

Rotahaler

Figure 2.2   How to use the Rotahaler
1 Hold the Rotahaler vertically and put capsule *coloured end uppermost* into the 'square' hole. Make sure top of Rotacap is level with top of hole. (If there is a Rotacap already in the device this will be pushed into the shell.)
2 Hold the Rotahaler horizontally and twist the barrel sharply forwards and backwards – this splits the capsule into two.
3 Breathe out gently. Keep the Rotahaler level and put the mouthpiece between your lips and teeth, and breathe in the powder quickly and deeply.
4 Remove the Rotahaler from your mouth and hold your breath for about 10 seconds.

Always discuss the use of your device with your doctor or asthma nurse.

change rapidly owing to sudden exposure to trigger factors (see Chapter 1). It is therefore important always to carry a reliever inhaler, such as Ventolin, with you.

My 4-year-old son has recently been diagnosed as having asthma. He has been prescribed Intal. What does this do?

Intal (sodium cromoglycate) is a drug which was developed from an Egyptian weed used to help people with asthma many centuries ago. It appears to have many actions, but the most important of these is that it can 'block' allergic reactions that take place in the eyes, nose or lungs. For example, someone with hay fever suffers from allergic reactions in the eyes and nose and, of course, in asthma allergic reactions occur in the lungs.

Sodium cromoglycate can be inhaled nasally, as Rynacrom, or used in eye drops, as Opticrom, for hay fever. Intal is the preparation for asthma.

It is a **preventive** treatment, which means it must be taken regularly, not just when there are symptoms. Intal is more effective in children than adults, particularly those in whom allergy is the most important trigger for their asthma. For constant protection Intal should be taken four times a day, although recent research suggests that once the asthma is well controlled this can be reduced to three times or even twice a day.

It is important to realize that Intal is a preventive treatment and will have no immediate effect on the relief of symptoms. However, it can be very effective if an extra dose is taken about 30 minutes before exposure to a known trigger, such as a pet, or before exercise.

Intal can be taken using the Spinhaler (dry powder capsules) or the pressurized (metered dose) inhaler, either on its own or through the Fisonair spacer (see the next section for more information about these devices). For very small children Intal can be given in a solution through a nebulizer. It is extremely safe, and there are virtually no side effects. Very occasionally the powder from the spincaps used in the Spinhaler can cause coughing and irritation of the airways.

What exactly does prednisolone do?

Prednisolone is a treatment which is taken by mouth. It is one of a group of drugs whose proper name is *corticosteroids*. We do not completely understand all of its actions in treating asthma. However, we do know that it reduces and dampens down inflammation dramatically. We also know that it reduces the swelling and secretions (phlegm) that are produced in the airways during acute asthma.

It is the most commonly prescribed oral steroid in the UK. It is often used to treat acute attacks of asthma and, less commonly, as long-term therapy for chronic severe asthma. In acute asthma, it is

important to make sure that a high enough dose is prescribed, and
that it is given for a long enough time for the inflammation to
subside. In an adult such a dose would usually be in the range of
30–60 milligrams per day, and for a child 20–30 milligrams per day.
It works better when the tablets are taken all together in one dose
(e.g. after breakfast) rather than in divided doses through the day.

There is a soluble form called Prednesol. This is extremely useful
for children, and for people who find tablets hard to swallow.
Prednisolone can also be given in a special coated form to reduce
the risk of indigestion and stomach ulcers, which otherwise can be
troublesome side effects. Taking the tablets with food, rather than
on an empty stomach, also reduces the risk of indigestion.

**Although I am currently on a high dose of inhaled steroids
(preventers), I have been using my reliever inhaler a lot
recently. My doctor says that I would need to use my reliever
inhaler much less if I started using a different inhaler called
salmeterol as well as my preventer. What is salmeterol, and
why is it different?**

Salmeterol xinafoate (brand name Serevent) and eformoterol
fumarate (brand name Foradil and Oxis) are long-acting inhaled
drugs belonging to the group of *beta agonist bronchodilators* (see
the **Glossary** for more details of this group of drugs). This means
they are related to the reliever treatments (such as Ventolin and
Bricanyl) with which we are familiar, but differ in that they
produce prolonged opening up of the airways, lasting for about 12
hours. They are usually taken twice daily, and are **not** intended for
immediate relief of symptoms. Serevent comes in either a standard pressurized inhaler, a Diskhaler or an Accuhaler. Foradil
comes as a dry powder capsule for use in a breath-actuated
inhaler. The effect is noticeable after 5–10 minutes, but the full
benefit is not generally noticed until after several doses of the
drug. Because of its long-lasting action, it can be particularly
useful in treating people who have night time symptoms.

Like preventers, they should be taken regularly to gain full
benefit. Salmeterol xinafoate and eformoterol fumarate are **not**
a replacement for, or an alternative to, inhaled steroids or other
preventive asthma treatments. They are regarded as additional

therapy, rather than a first-line treatment, if usual doses of preventer are not controlling asthma. It is very important that
inhaled steroids or other preventive treatments are not stopped
when salmeterol or eformoterol are prescribed. Many people
notice that they need little, or none, of their short-acting relieving treatment once they start taking one of these long-acting
bronchodilators.

**What is cyclosporin? Why are we not using it to treat asthma
yet?**

Cyclosporin is a very powerful and expensive drug that works by
reducing the body's response to inflammation, which may be
caused by a number of problems. For example, it is used for
treating people with cancer, or people who have had transplants.
It is known as an 'immunosuppressive' drug, because it dampens
down (suppresses) the body's immune system which protects
against infections.

Because it works against inflammation, it has been used in
experimental trials in severely affected people whose asthma
cannot be controlled with the usual asthma drugs. The results
showed some very encouraging responses in some people, suggesting that this may be a type of drug to prove helpful in future
treatment of asthma. Methotrexate is another powerful drug with
anti-inflammatory effects which has sometimes been used for
severe asthma.

Both of these drugs have potentially severe side effects which
rule them out for treating mild or moderate asthma. For cyclosporin, apart from suppressing the body's own immune system
(which can lead to severe infections), these include anaemia,
kidney damage, rashes and severe overgrowth of body hair. So,
even though it seems to be very effective, it is too toxic to
recommend for routine use. The exciting prospect for the future is
that less powerful but more effective drugs may be developed
using cyclosporin as the starting point.

**Why won't my GP prescribe antibiotics to have at home to
be taken at the first sign of a chest infection? This form
of treatment meant less time off work for me, and**

**consequently less pressure from my employers, which
itself tends to make my asthma worse.**

This is a rather tricky question which, without knowing your
individual details, we will have to answer in general terms. The
difficulty arises in having to distinguish between asthma and a
true chest infection. Although antibiotics may help to clear a chest
infection rapidly, they are not often helpful in the treatment of
asthma. Although asthma is often triggered by an infection, such
as the common cold, this infection is nearly always caused by a
virus. Viruses are not affected at all by antibiotics, so there is no
point giving them for virus infections.

The symptoms of an asthma attack may resemble a chest
infection, with coughing, wheezing and shortness of breath.
Asthma may also cause you to cough up lots of phlegm – leading to
the false impression that your symptoms are due to an infection
which needs antibiotics.

It is usually much better for you to increase your asthma medication at the start of these symptoms. Then only if they do not improve
should you consult your doctor to see if an antibiotic is needed.

**Are there particular times of the day when medication
should be taken, or should I leave it as long as possible
before taking it?**

The answer to this depends on the medication you are taking.
Inhaled steroids (Becotide, Becloforte, Pulmicort, Aerobec,
Flixotide) are usually taken twice daily. The actual time does not
matter, but it is useful to take them night and morning, before
brushing your teeth. This makes it part of a routine, but also
ensures that you rinse your mouth out afterwards. This reduces
the chance of side effects, especially *thrush* in the throat. The
other preventers (Intal, Tilade) are usually prescribed two to four
times daily, at least initially. As long as these are reasonably
spread through the day, they do not need to be taken at particular
times. However, as with inhaled steroids, it is good to get into a
routine. The benefit from preventer treatments comes from taking
them regularly, and to do this it is best to have a routine.

Reliever treatments such as Ventolin, Aerolin, Airomir

(salbutamol) or Bricanyl (terbutaline) should be taken when you feel wheezy or short of breath, or if you feel an attack coming on – there are no set times for these.

Serevent (salmeterol xinafoate) and Foradil and Oxis (eformoterol fumarate) belong to a class of bronchodilator treatments which have a long action of 10–12 hours. They should be taken regularly, twice daily.

As you can see, you don't have to be rigid in the times when you take your medication. However, we do not advise you to leave it as long as possible before you take it as there are no benefits to be gained from unnecessary delay.

Should I have an anti-'flu injection?

If you are prone to bad attacks of asthma during the winter months, the answer is yes.

Virus infections are important triggers for asthma in many people. Influenza (better known as 'flu) is one such virus infection. It can cause serious pneumonia, particularly in elderly people or those with chronic chest trouble. For people with asthma, 'flu may bring on a severe episode of asthma. It is generally recommended that all these people should have protection against 'flu. This is also recommended by the Department of Health.

An anti-'flu injection once a year will help to prevent the illness, or at least reduce its severity. There are few side effects from this injection. Some people are unlucky, and they suffer from a mild 'flu-like illness for a few days after the injection. A prescription is required, but many general practitioners dispense 'flu vaccine, in which case it is free to their patients. Those who are exempt from prescription charges do not pay in any case.

Is it alright to use eye drops as well as inhalers?

It may seem extremely strange but certain eye drops, prescribed for the condition glaucoma, may aggravate asthma. Timoptol is the most important of these. It is a beta blocker, which means it has the opposite effect to the (beta stimulant) action of the reliever inhalers. Even minuscule doses of these eye drops absorbed into the system have been known to have a bad effect on asthma. Most other types of eye drops used for glaucoma cause no problems. If you are unlucky enough to have both glaucoma and asthma, you should discuss this problem with your doctor.

Devices

What is the difference between the various puffers you can use?

There is quite a range of inhaler devices (*puffers*) for the treatment of asthma, and you will find illustrations of all of them in this section. It is important to select the right one for each individual, as the wrong choice of device is often the only reason why someone's asthma gets out of control.

The pressurised aerosol (metered dose) inhaler (Figure 2.3) is still the most commonly used device, and this is the type commonly known as the 'puffer'. It does have disadvantages, the most important one being that a lot of people find the technique difficult. A number of surveys have shown that many of those using aerosol inhalers use them incorrectly. The chief problem is that very good co-ordination is needed during the breathing in of the drug, and this is difficult to achieve without careful practice.

The Autohaler (Figure 2.4,) and Easi-Breathe (Figure 2.5), overcome co-ordination problems by releasing the drug automatically as you breathe in through the mouthpiece.

Devices that give the drug in the form of dry powder do not require co-ordination by the patient. Some of these devices, such as the Spinhaler (for Intal – Figure 2.6) and the Rotahaler (for Ventolin and Becotide – Figure 2.2), require the storage of capsules which may be affected by the atmosphere and which can be fiddly to use, especially for elderly patients. The Diskhaler (for Ventolin, Becotide, Becloforte, Flixotide and Serevent – Figure 2.1) has a set number of doses of powdered medicine set into a circular disk protected by thin foil. The disk is slotted into the device itself. Flixotide, Serevent and Ventolin are now available in an Accuhaler (see Figure 2.7), a multi-dose dry powder device with a counter.

The Turbohaler (for Bricanyl and Pulmicort – Figure 2.8) has either 50, 100 or 200 pre-packed doses available inside the device.

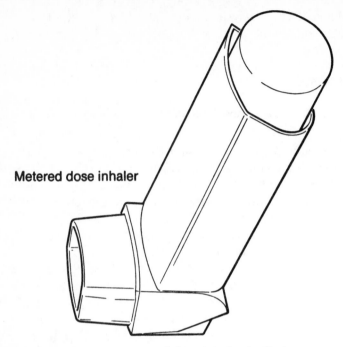

Metered dose inhaler

Figure 2.3   How to use a metered dose inhaler (puffer)
1 Remove the cap and shake the inhaler.
2 Breathe out gently.
3 Put the mouthpiece in your mouth and at the start of inspiration (breathing in), which should be slow and deep, press the canister down and continue to inhale (breathe in) deeply.
4 Hold your breath for about 10 seconds, or for as long as possible.
5 Wait about 30 seconds before taking another inhalation.

Always discuss the use of your device with your doctor or asthma nurse.

An indication is given when only 20 doses remain in the device, but otherwise it is difficult to tell how many doses have been taken. Pulmicort (budesonide) is available in an aerosol (pressurized inhaler) and a dry powder inhaler (Turbohaler). The Turbohaler is twice as effective as the aerosol inhaler for budesonide. Therefore your doctor will usually prescribe half the dose when switching someone from an aerosol to a Turbohaler.

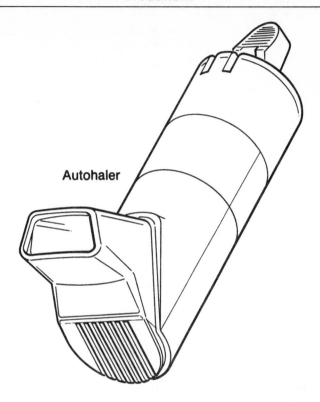

Autohaler

Figure 2.4 How to use the Autohaler
1 Remove the protective mouthpiece and shake the inhaler.
2 Hold the inhaler upright and push the lever right up.
3 Breathe out gently. Keep the inhaler upright and put the mouthpiece in your mouth and close your lips around it. (The air holes must not be blocked by your hand.)
4 Breathe in steadily through your mouth. DON'T stop breathing when the inhaler 'clicks' but continue taking a really deep breath.
5 Hold your breath for about 10 seconds.

NB The lever must be pushed up ('on') before each dose and pushed down ('off') again afterwards, otherwise it will not operate.
Always discuss the use of your device with your doctor or asthma nurse.

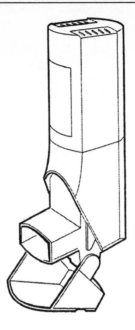

Figure 2.5   How to use the Easi-Breathe
1 Shake inhaler.
2 Hold inhaler upright. Open the cap.
3 Breathe out gently. Keep inhaler upright, put mouthpiece in mouth and close lips and teeth around it (the air holes on the top must not be blocked by the hand).
4 Breathe in steadily through the mouthpiece. Don't stop breathing when the inhaler 'puffs' and continue taking a really deep breath.
5 Hold breath for about 10 seconds.
6 After use, hold inhaler upright and immediately close cap.
7 For a second dose, wait a few seconds before repeating sections 1–6.

Always demonstrate to the patient how to use the Easi-Breathe

Are inhalers the most effective way for me to take my anti-asthma treatment?

Generally, yes. The aim of asthma treatment is to achieve maximum control of symptoms with the minimum amount of medi-

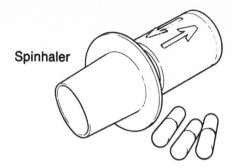

Figure 2.6   How to use the Spinhaler
1 Hold the Spinhaler upright, with the mouthpiece downwards, and unscrew the body.
2 Put *coloured* end of the spincap into *cup* of propeller.
3 Screw the two parts together and move grey sleeve up and down once or twice – this will pierce the capsule.
4 Breathe out gently, put the Spinhaler into your mouth so your lips touch the flange, and breathe in quickly and deeply.
5 Remove the Spinhaler from your mouth. Hold your breath for about 10 seconds and then breathe out slowly.
6 If any powder is left in the spincap, repeat steps 4 and 5 until it is empty.

Always discuss the use of your device with your doctor or asthma nurse.

cation. The great advantage of inhaling your treatment is that only a tiny dose of the drug needs to be prescribed, because the drug is delivered directly to your lungs. This dose works faster, and there is less chance of you developing side effects.

However, the choice of inhaler device is almost as important as the choice of drug to be delivered. There are many different devices available, and unless the right one is selected, much of the drug will be wasted. Selecting the wrong device or poor use of the right device is frequently the only reason why people find their asthma getting out of control.

I don't like the taste of inhalers, what else could I use?

This can be a difficult problem. Sometimes it is the taste of the propellant for the aerosol that people do not like, and this may be

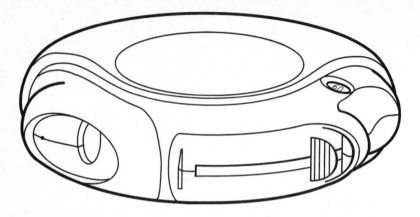

Figure 2.7   How to use the Accuhaler

1 Hold the outer casing of the Accuhaler in one hand whilst pushing the thumbgrip away until a click is heard.
2 Hold the device with the mouthpiece towards you, slide the lever away until it clicks. This makes the dose available for inhalation and moves the dose counter on.
3 Holding the device level, breathe out gently away from the device, put the mouthpiece in the mouth and suck in steadily and deeply.
4 Remove the device from the mouth and hold your breath for about 10 seconds.
5 To close, slide the thumbgrip back towards you as far as it will go, until it clicks.
6 For a second dose, repeat sections 1–5.

Always ask your doctor or asthma nurse to demonstrate how to use the Accuhaler.

the case for you. If so, a switch to one of the dry powder inhaler devices (Diskhaler, Rotahaler, Accuhaler, Turbohaler or Click-haler – Figures 2.1, 2.2, 2.7, 2.8, 2.9) might help you. In some of these there is a sweet tasting lactose powder that many people prefer.

So far there is no alternative to inhaled treatment which can be as effective, and yet be given in such low dosages. Although it would be possible for you to take tablets, inevitably these would have to be given in much higher doses to have the same

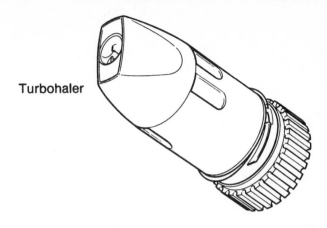

Turbohaler

Figure 2.8   How to use the Turbohaler
1 Unscrew and lift off the white cover. Hold the Turbohaler upright and twist the grip forwards and backwards as far as it will go. You should hear a click.
2 Breathe out gently, put the mouthpiece between your lips and breathe in as deeply as possible. Even when a full dose is taken there may be no taste.
3 Remove the Turbohaler from your mouth and hold your breath for about 10 seconds. Replace the white cover.

Always discuss the use of your device with your doctor or asthma nurse.

effect as the inhaled version of the drug. So you wouldn't get the taste problem, but you would be more likely to get other side effects.

In practice, not all inhaled medications have the same taste, and for most people they have no taste at all. It could just be that you have been unlucky in the particular sort prescribed for you. One particular treatment was known to have an unpleasant taste, but this has now been re-formulated to have quite a pleasant mint flavour, and this has largely overcome the problem. We suggest it would be worth talking to your doctor or asthma nurse about your treatment. It may be possible to change your inhalers, but you do need to be sure that you are receiving the right treatment.

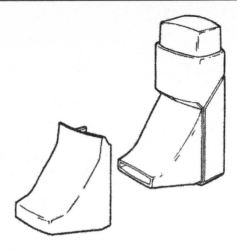

Figure 2.9   How to use the Clickhaler
 1 Hold Clickhaler upright.
 2 Remove mouthpiece from inhaler.
 3 Shake inhaler.
 4 Continue to hold Clickhaler upright with your thumb on base and a
    finger on coloured push button.
 5 Press dosing button down firmly – once only, then release.
 6 Breathe out gently and put mouthpiece between lips and teeth,
    sealing lips around mouthpiece (do not breathe out into Clickhaler).
 7 Breathe in steadily and deeply. Remove Clickhaler from mouth and
    hold breath for about 5–10 seconds. Breathe out slowly.
 8 For a second dose, keep Clickhaler upright and repeat steps 3–7.
 9 Replace mouthpiece cover after use.
10 There is a dose counter at the back of inhaler. After 190 actuations a
    red warning appears in the counter window which shows there are
    10 actuations left. When no actuations are left, the inhaler locks and
    can no longer be used, and should be discarded.

Always demonstrate to the patient how to use the Clickhaler

**Sometimes when I use my inhaler I think I haven't used it
properly. Should I repeat the dose?**

No, not necessarily. There could be two reasons why you are not
using your inhaler properly. The first could be that you are getting

your co-ordination wrong, so that you are not breathing in at the same time as the drug is released from the inhaler. If this happens, the treatment ends up in your mouth or nose, and doesn't get into your lungs, where it is needed. This is particularly likely to happen with a metered dose inhaler (or 'puffer' – Figure 2.3), because it is often quite difficult to get the co-ordination exactly right.

The second reason could be that you find it harder to use your inhaler properly when your asthma is bad. This is because it is more difficult to breathe in fully if your airways are narrowed. This second reason is more common than is realized, but in both cases we would suggest that you need to ask for advice. If you are using the inhaler incorrectly, you might be helped by a change to a different device which is triggered simply by the effort of breathing. There are several of these so called *breath-actuated* devices, including dry powder devices (Spinhaler, Rotahaler, Diskhaler, Accuhaler, Turbohaler, Clickhaler – Figures 2.1, 2.2, 2.6–2.9), Autohaler and Easi-Breathe (Figures 2.4, 2.5). A further advantage of the dry powder devices is that is possible for you to see whether all the powder has been used after you have taken your dose.

If you notice a problem only when your asthma is bad, then a spacer device (such as an Able Spacer; Aerochamber; Volumatic – Figure 2.10; or a Nebuhaler – Figure 2.11) could be useful. With the spacer you need only to breathe in and out gently (called *tidal breathing*), rather than sucking in deeply. Because of this, spacers are often used during acute attacks, and can be as effective as nebulizers. We discuss spacer devices in more detail later in this section.

Why is my friend on a different kind of inhaler?

There could be several reasons. The most likely is that yours has been selected by your doctor or asthma nurse because it is the most suitable one for you. At present there are around 15 different inhaler devices available in the UK. They all deliver the same types of treatments, but do so in different ways. The metered dose inhaler (commonly known as the 'puffer') is still the most commonly prescribed. Many people have difficulty with it because they can't co-ordinate their breathing in with the release of the spray in

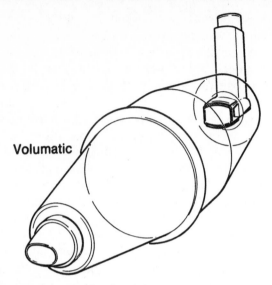

Volumatic

Figure 2.10   How to use the Volumatic spacer device
1 Remove the cap, shake the inhaler and insert into the device.
2 Place the mouthpiece in your mouth.
3 Press the canister once to release a dose of the drug.
4 Take a slow, deep breath in.
5 Hold your breath for about 10 seconds, then breathe out through the mouthpiece.
6 Breathe in again but do not press the canister.
7 Remove the device from your mouth.
8 Wait about 30 seconds before taking a second dose.
9 Leave to dry after washing – never wipe dry.

order to use it effectively. Most of the newer devices (such as the Autohaler or Easi-Breathe, and all the dry powder devices – Figures 2.1, 2.2, 2.4–2.8) do not require such good co-ordination, and so are easier to use correctly. They are particularly useful for children and the elderly. Your nurses and doctors should help you to find the type of device which suits you best. After all, you are the person who has to take the treatment, and so you need to be happy with the device. What suits one person will not suit another, so there is no reason why your friend should not be on a different inhaler.

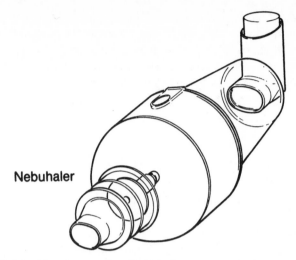

Nebuhaler

Figure 2.11   How to use the Nebuhaler spacer device to give asthma
treatments to young children
1 Remove the cap, shake the inhaler and insert into the device.
2 Place the mouthpiece in the child's mouth (be careful that the child's
  lips are *behind* the ring).
3 Seal the child's lips round the mouthpiece by gently placing the fin-
  gers of one hand round the lips.
4 Encourage the child to breathe in and out slowly and gently. (This will
  make a 'clicking' sound as the valve opens and closes.)
5 Once the breathing pattern is well established, depress the canister
  with your free hand and leave the device in the same position as the
  child continues to breathe (called tidal breathing) several more times.
6 Remove the device from the child's mouth.
7 Leave to dry after washing – never wipe dry.

Can I let my daughter play with the device in order to get familiar with it?

As long as she is supervised, and cannot take several doses of a drug,
this is a very sensible suggestion on two counts. Firstly, it can help
your doctor or asthma nurse choose the right device for your
daughter. However, it is important not to offer her all the available
devices to play with, as some are unsuitable for young children.
Secondly, there is no doubt that the more familiar your child is with her

device, the more likely she is to use it effectively. We often recommend that not only should the **child** play with the device, but that they should watch one of their **parents** use it as well. This undoubtedly makes a child feel less worried. If you ask your doctor or nurse they may be able to provide you with a dummy (placebo) device. These can be very useful for practice and play. If your daughter is prescribed one of the large spacer devices, try decorating it with coloured stickers of her choice – this can certainly brighten up treatment times.

How can I tell when my daughter's MDI (metered dose inhaler, or puffer) is running low?

Shaking the MDI can give an idea as to how full it is. This is sometimes difficult. Although not recommended by the manufacturers, as a last resort, you could drop the aerosol (after removing it from its plastic holder) into a bowl of water and then judge how full it is by the way it floats.

If this problem really bothers you there are alternative devices, mainly dry powder ones (Diskhaler, Rotahaler, Spinhaler, Accuhaler, Turbohaler – Figures 2.1, 2.2, 2.6–2.8), which would give you some indication of how many doses of her treatment your daughter had remaining.

It is sensible always to have a spare inhaler available. Most doctors do not mind prescribing an extra inhaler as a spare, but they are very expensive, and spares should be kept in a safe place. Put in a request for a replacement inhaler when the spare is used for the first time. This advice is very relevant for people going away from home.

Can I get another device from my doctor if I am not happy with my present inhaler?

Yes, of course. There is quite a wide range of inhaler devices now available for asthma treatment, so it is not necessary to persist for months or years with a device, if you just cannot get on with it. The best approach would be to book an appointment with the asthma clinic, if there is one at your doctor's practice. Failing that, book an appointment with your doctor, practice nurse or pharmacist. Many surgeries keep a selection of the inhaler devices, so that you can try them out. Once you have agreed on which device suits you best, then you can change to that for your regular prescription.

Where can I go to get someone to show me how to use the inhaler properly?

There are quite a few places where you can get assistance with this problem. An asthma clinic at your own GP's practice would be ideal. Although many practices do have such clinics running, not all do. In this case, your GP or practice nurse should still be able to help. Your local pharmacist may also be able to give you a leaflet and some practical guidance.

In a few parts of the country, asthma centres are being established within communities or districts so that local people can call in to get advice and sort out this kind of problem. These may become more widespread in the next few years. Finally, branches of the National Asthma Campaign (see Appendix), which exist all over the UK, have a number of members who are very experienced in the practicalities of looking after asthma.

So, you have a number of choices, but make sure you do go for one of them!

Are all people with asthma treated the same?

No. People are individuals and asthma affects everyone in a different way. The basic principles of treatment are applied to people with asthma in different ways. For example, severity obviously determines the type and dose (amount) of drug prescribed.

Self-help in asthma care is encouraged and taught by many doctors and nurses. However, individual people differ in their desire and ability to take responsibility for the management of their own illness. It can be as wrong to force someone to become self-reliant as to stop it in someone who wants that independence.

There are many inhaler devices available for delivery of asthma drugs. This is because people differ in their ability to use devices, and it is a good idea for practices and clinics to have a range, so that everyone can find the device that suits them best. For example there are devices specially designed for very young or elderly people. Some have been adapted for use by people with arthritis. These include the Haleraid (for Ventolin or Becotide) which is on sale by retail pharmacies, and the Turbohaler arthritis aid, available free from Astra Pharmaceuticals, supplied on request to the medical profession.

In asthma, the method of delivering inhalers is very inconvenient – isn't there a medicine I could take instead?

Not all inhalers are inconvenient, in fact the latest inhaler devices which have been introduced are compact, convenient and very easy to use.

The Diskhaler (Figure 2.1), the Turbohaler (Figure 2.8), the Autohaler (Figure 2.4), Easi-Breathe (Figure 2.5), Clickhaler (Figure 2.9) and Accuhaler (Figure 2.7) are all extremely portable and can be used by most age groups with only a minimal amount of instruction required. Also, inhalers are the most effective way for you to take your treatment – see the answer to the next question for the reasons why.

Why use the inhaler when the syrup is easier to dispense?

You are right – swallowing a spoonful of medicine is easier than using an inhaler device correctly. Why then do we, wherever possible, recommend that you inhale your treatment?

Swallowed medications – and this includes tablets and capsules as well as syrup – are taken up into the bloodstream and circulate all round the body. Because of this they do not act on the airways anything like as quickly as drugs delivered by inhaler devices. Also, as one might expect, a much larger dose is needed in order to be effective.

The treatment most likely to be prescribed in syrup or tablet form is one of the reliever drugs, such as salbutamol (Ventolin or Volmax), terbutaline (Bricanyl syrup) or bambuterol (Bambec). When dispensed in this way, these drugs quite frequently cause side effects. The main side effects are pounding of the heart, and shaking or trembling of the hands. Xanthine bronchodilators, such as *aminophylline* (Phyllocontin) or *theophylline* (Uniphyllin) may be prescribed in syrup or tablet form. These can also cause unpleasant side effects such as indigestion, nausea, palpitations and difficulty with sleeping.

Side effects with inhaled treatments are much milder and occur much less frequently. Much smaller doses of inhaled drug can be given with better effect, and the risk of side effects is much lower.

Who will benefit from the new tablet treatments for asthma?

Tablets are not new in asthma treatment. Inhalers have always been regarded as the best treatment for asthma because the drug is delivered directly to the lungs where it is expected to work. Tablets have therefore been used only in people unable to use inhalers. One type of tablet, the xanthine group of drugs, are used in people with more severe asthma in addition to high doses of inhaled steroids and long-acting relievers. Recently, the xanthines (Phyllocontin Continuus, Nuelin, Slophyllin, Theo-Dur, Uni-phyllin) have been used, to a lesser extent in the UK, in low doses in addition to low dose inhaled steroids in some patients. Some of the relievers are also available in tablets: salbutamol (Volmax), bambuterol (Bambec), orciprenaline (Alupent).

Two new asthma tablets, which are anti-inflammatory drugs (preventers), have recently been licensed for use in asthma in the UK. These are called Singulair (montelukast) and Accolate (zafirlukast) and are anti-inflammatory (i.e. preventer) drugs. They are the first new group of asthma drugs to be developed for many years. At present these drugs are mainly prescribed to be used in addition to inhaled steroids, although Accolate (zafir-lukast) has been granted a licence for prescription on its own. These drugs seem to improve symptoms of asthma in some people not afforded relief from the inhaled steroids and bronchodilators drugs (relievers). So they seem to work in a different way from the other preventers. Side effects include mainly headaches and tummy upsets.

These drugs may be particularly helpful in asthma sufferers who are allergic to aspirin.

The launch of leukotiene receptor antagonists (LTRAs) in the USA has resulted in a controversy. Churg–Strauss syndrome is a condition that may be confused with asthma. Many of these patients' symptoms are well controlled on cortisone (steroids) tablets. When the LTRAs came onto the market, in the USA, many doctors tried to replace the cortisone tablets (or to reduce the dose) in more severe asthmatic people by prescribing these new

LTRA drugs. As a result many new cases of Churg–Strauss were diagnosed. There is considerable debate whether the LTRAs 'unmasked' or caused these cases of Churg–Strauss syndrome.

What can I, as a mother, do to help give my baby asthma drugs?

Babies of under a year old are notoriously difficult to treat. This is not only because they often don't respond to the conventional first line treatment of relievers (such as Ventolin Evohaler, Bricanyl or Atrovent), but also because it is difficult to deliver any of the drugs easily to the baby's airways. We suggest that you do persevere with the asthma drugs which your doctor has prescribed and recommend that if possible you give the treatment using a spacer device.

Some of these devices (e.g. Aerochamber and Babyhaler) have masks attached, and can be used effectively for very young babies. Masks may be attached to the other types of spacer (Volumatic, Nebuhaler, Able Spacer, Fisonair). Your baby can be held in your arms, but for preference should be lying down. The Nebuhaler or Volumatic should be tilted vertically so that the aerosol canister is higher than the mask (Figure 2.12). In this position the valve remains open all the time. When the mask is in position over the baby's mouth and nose, the canister should be triggered; the drug is sprayed through the device to the mask and your baby inhales it. There is no seal between the mask and your baby's face – we find that usually babies are blissfully unaware they are receiving any treatment! Inevitably some of the drug will escape into the atmosphere rather than going into your baby's lungs but this does not matter.

What are the benefits of using a Volumatic?

A Volumatic (Figure 2.10) is an example of a large spacer device designed to ease the use of certain inhaled drugs. The Nebuhaler (Figure 2.11) is very similar in appearance and action, and the Integra is an integral compact spacer device containing Becloforte. The Aerochamber can take any of the metered dose inhalers.

There are three main advantages of using these devices.

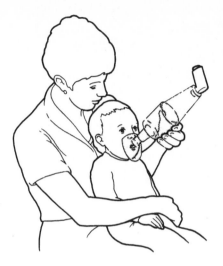

Figure 2.12 A spacer device fitted with a face mask can be used to give asthma treatment to a baby.

- They are easier to use effectively than conventional aerosol inhalers and they are almost as effective as a nebulizer.
- More drug gets into the lungs, where it is needed.
- There is less chance of side effects. With ordinary inhalers, a lot of the drug ends up in the mouth where it is swallowed and absorbed into the blood, and this may lead to side effects. The use of the Volumatic, the Nebuhaler, the Aerochamber, the Able Spacer, and the Integra reduces the risk of these.

Can I use Ventolin Evohaler, Becotide and Intal in my Volumatic?

Your Ventolin Evohaler and Becotide (along with Becloforte and Serevent) fit the Volumatic (Figure 2.10) which is made by Allen & Hanburys Ltd. Intal (and Tilade) fit the Fisonair which is made by Aventis. Tilade also comes in the Syncroner. As you can see the manufacturers of the treatments make their own special devices to use with their treatments. In addition, AstraZeneca, who manufacture Bricanyl and Pulmicort, make the Nebuhaler spacer device (Figure 2.11) for which there is a special adaptor for the

use of Intal. The Integra, made by Allen & Hanburys Ltd, contains
only Becloforte.

What is a nebulizer?

A nebulizer (Figure 2.13) breaks up liquid drugs into tiny droplets,
forming a mist which you can then breathe into your lungs.

Many people with asthma feel that a nebulizer is some kind of
magical device. We understand why this view arises, and indeed
the nebulizer is a marvellous piece of equipment. However, it is
important to be aware that the nebulizer is no more than a very
effective way of giving standard asthma treatments. The Aerochamber and AbleSpacer can be used with any of the puffers. In

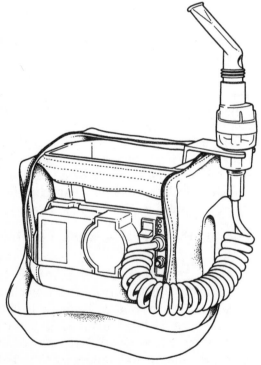

Figure 2.13 The Medic-Aid Freeway Lite Nebuliser-Compressor,
which is one of the various types of nebulizer available.

fact, experts are now advising that a spacer with a puffer should be used instead of a nebulizer.

There are two sorts in current use – the jet nebulizer and the ultrasonic nebulizer. The jet nebulizer is electrically powered (except for one model which uses a foot pump). It works by a stream of compressed air or oxygen being forced through a fine nozzle into a nebulizing chamber. The drug solution is drawn up into the chamber and broken into particles of mist. You inhale the tiny particles, while the larger droplets fall back to the bottom of the chamber and are then re-nebulised.

Ultrasonic nebulizers work in a different way, although the end result – the aerosol mist – is identical. Ultrasound waves break up the drug solution into a spray formation. These nebulizers are completely silent when in operation and the mist is triggered only when you breathe in. This means that no drug is wasted and you can have a rest without switching the machine off. Elderly people often find this the ideal system. We have found, however, that it is not suitable for the regular administration of preventive drugs to small children because they do not have enough co-ordination to trigger the mist.

Most people would agree that, if a nebulizer really is needed, the electrically powered jet nebulizers are the first choice for anyone – young or old – who requires home nebulization. They are noisy, but they cost much less, and are easy to use.

Don't go out and buy a nebulizer without discussing it carefully with your doctor.

Wouldn't it be better to use the nebulizer the whole time?

Long-term, regular nebulization should be needed only by a very small percentage of people with asthma. These are usually people with chronic asthma who need very high doses of reliever treatment, or young children who cannot manage any other sort of inhaler device. For other people it would be a waste of time (and money) to use a nebulizer in this way. It takes about 10 minutes to use a nebulizer, compared with the seconds required to use an inhaler. It needs to be plugged into a power point and your mobility can be very much reduced by this requirement. Another difficulty is that the dose given by a nebulizer is anything from 10 to 50 times higher than a normal dose through an inhaler, and this can cause problems with side effects. Some people do place too much faith in nebulizers, and they expect miracles. In fact too much confidence in nebulizers may lead to a dangerous delay in seeking medical advice when asthma is bad. For this reason in particular we do not recommend that you purchase a nebulizer without clear advice and approval from your doctor.

Should we buy our own nebulizer?

Obviously we can't give you a definite answer without knowing your exact circumstances, but nebulizers (Figure 2.13) are generally used in one or more of three situations. We need to look at these separately, because it makes a difference as to whether or not you should consider buying one.

- **Emergency treatment.** High dose reliever treatments usually give rapid relief during acute asthma attacks, and a nebulizer or a spacer is a very good way of giving this. A few people have asthma that gets worse so quickly that they need to have a nebulizer to hand. For them, it is very valuable to have their own nebulizer. The vast majority, however, do not have asthma that is so severe, and they can take steps to control a worsening situation without requiring a home nebulizer.
- **People with asthma unable to use inhaler devices.** Very young children, and the elderly or infirm may be unable to use any other sort of inhaler device effectively. In these cases, a nebulizer may be required. In young children they are used mainly for giving the preventive treatments regularly, and so it can be very useful to own one. Nowadays, the range of inhaler devices and spacers is so wide that it is becoming more and more unusual to find anyone who cannot manage at least one.
- **Severe chronic asthma.** A few people (usually elderly) need regular high dose reliever treatment. They have very severe obstruction of their airways, and sometimes need oxygen to be kept in the home. The nebulizer can be used three or four times a day, and give much relief.

In some cases, nebulizers may be borrowed long term from hospitals or health authorities. Buying a nebulizer yourself can be fairly costly. Whatever the circumstances, do not buy a home nebulizer without a full discussion with your doctor.

Can I buy my own nebulizer? And if so, how do I get one?

The first part of this question, which seems simple enough, is not always an easy one to answer. Anyone **can** buy a nebulizer but always the more important question is '**should** I buy my own nebulizer?' For the answer to that, please see the previous question.

Before you embark on any purchase you need to establish with your doctor whether it is right for you to have one. Whilst the idea of home nebulizers may be attractive, it is vital to appreciate that they can be dangerous if not used with the right safeguards. This involves knowing how often to use the nebulizer for emergency purposes, and also how to measure your response to it. More often, nebulizers are needed for the regular giving of preventer drugs to children. In these cases the nebulizer is not dangerous but it may be unnecessary as there are other simpler ways of giving the same drug (for example, a spacer used with a puffer).

If, however, you do need a nebulizer to take your treatment then it is likely that you will have to pay for it. Nebulizers cannot be prescribed on the NHS in the same way as spacer devices (e.g. Volumatic, Nebuhaler or Aerochamber – Figures 2.10 and 2.11) can be, but many hospitals have a number of machines that they will lend, or even give, to patients. Nebulizers powered by electric compressors are the most popular but are quite costly, but it is possible to buy a foot pump nebulizer (based on the car tyre foot pump) which is much cheaper). If you have an asthma attack, someone else will need to operate the foot pump for you!

If your doctor has agreed that it is right for you to have your own nebulizer, you will be able to get VAT exemption on the purchase price if your order is accompanied by a letter from your doctor.

There are many different manufacturers of nebulizers: your doctor or asthma nurse should be able to provide you with the names. You can order direct from the manufacturer. Whichever model you choose, you will generally be supplied with all the accessories you need, including the compressor, nebulizer chamber, mask or mouthpiece and plastic tubing.

My neighbour's son has a nebulizer. My daughter now has asthma. Should we borrow the nebulizer if we run into trouble?

In an emergency, while you are waiting for medical assistance to arrive, this would probably be a sensible thing to do, but you should not rely on it as your stand-by. Nebulizers (Figure 2.13) are not the only method of treatment for uncontrolled asthma. They simply provide one method of delivering drugs into the lungs. It **is** a very good method, but is usually not necessary. As we have explained in preceding questions, the situations in which nebulizers are needed are:

- in very young children who cannot manage to use other types of device;
- in adults with severe chronic asthma who need very high doses of reliever treatment, often combined with oxygen;
- in emergencies when a person with acute asthma is too breathless to use their usual device.

If a nebulizer is not available, reliever drugs can be given through a spacer device such as a Volumatic, a Nebuhaler or an Aerochamber, and you might wish to talk to your doctor about having one of these. In real emergencies a spacer device can be made by making a hole for the inhaler mouthpiece in the bottom of a disposable plastic cup, such as a coffee or cola cup (see Figure 2.14). The emergency dose of reliever drug by any of these methods is between 15 and 30 puffs. You would need to give one puff of the drug every 10 seconds or so until your daughter started to improve.

How should I dispose of empty inhaler canisters?

Pressurized aerosol canisters should be treated like any other pressurized aerosols – for example like empty canisters of hairspray, deodorant or air freshener. They are all potentially hazardous if disposed of carelessly, so use common sense in getting rid of them carefully. They must not be thrown on to a fire (because they could explode), but they can be put out with your domestic rubbish. Non-pressurized inhaler devices pose no danger, and can

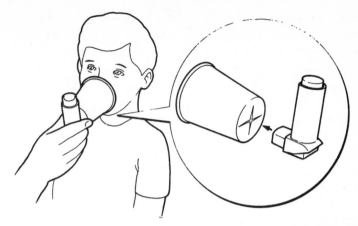

Figure 2.14   A paper or plastic coffee cup can be used to make an emergency spacer device to give a reliever inhaler to someone having an attack. The inhaler is pushed into a hole cut in the bottom of the cup. One puff every 10 seconds is used until the person is better.

also be put out with your other rubbish, but do make sure that they are empty. Supplies of unused drugs should always be returned to your pharmacist or doctor for safe disposal.

Side effects

How can long-term complications of treatments be balanced against the short-term benefits that they give?

There is no doubt that asthma causes considerable suffering. Many studies have confirmed this. However, many people do not realize the extent to which asthma is interfering with their lives. Approximately half of 61 000 people responding to a national survey reported that they had symptoms from asthma every day of their lives. Most of these simply accepted that such symptoms are part of life, and put up with the problems caused by them. This need not be the case with present day treatments. The short-term benefits of asthma treatment, improving the quality of life of many people, are immense.

It is always difficult to balance what gives pleasure today

against the problems that may occur in the future (a good example of this is cigarette smoking). Your question suggests that this balance needs to be made in asthma, and we agree. You may have to balance the 'pleasure' of no symptoms today, by taking treatment, against possible long-term side effects of that treatment. On the other hand you may feel that you prefer to take no treatment, and run the risk of dangerous attacks at any time, and long-term damage to your lungs later in life. This can be a difficult decision to take, and you should have every help from your medical advisers to let you decide what is the right course.

We consider that the evidence is strongly in favour of long-term safety of the drugs we use today, in inhaled form and in standard dosages. That is why **we** believe the advantages of short- and long-term treatment **outweigh considerably** any possible long-term complications of treatment. This is such an important issue for all asthmatics that we urge you to discuss it with all those involved in your asthma care.

What are the side effects of inhaled relievers?

All of the side effects with relievers are temporary, and occur only while the drug is being taken. It will depend on which relievers you are taking as to what the side effects – if any – might be. If you are taking relievers by inhaler and in normal doses, then very few side effects are likely. Any that you notice will be only temporary rather than long term. Relievers such as salbutamol (Ventolin), terbutaline sulphate (Bricanyl), and the longer acting drugs salmeterol (Serevent) and eformoterol fumarate (Foradil and Oxis) can cause a fine trembling of the muscles, particularly in the hands. This side effect usually wears off within a few minutes, or hours at most. If higher doses of these drugs are used, the pulse rate may increase, and palpitations, or pounding, of the heart may be noticed. This is not harmful but may be an unpleasant sensation.

Another group of relievers, called anticholinergic drugs, work in a different way, and tend to have different side effects. The best known of this group are ipratropium bromide (Atrovent) and oxitropium (Oxivent). Again, the side effects are very few with normal doses, but will increase with higher doses, particularly in nebulizer form. People prescribed these drugs may notice that their mouths become dry, and their vision blurred. Rarely, it may be difficult to pass urine, and constipation may occur.

Ventolin appears to work instantly for me, but what tissue damage is occurring?

None. On its own Ventolin is simply a reliever drug. This means that it opens up tightened airways. It **should** work instantly, and this relief should last at least four hours. It is suitable treatment for people with very mild asthma who only need relief medication occasionally.

The current advice is that, preferably, Ventolin should not be used regularly. This drug (as well as Bricanyl and other inhaled relievers) should only be used when you have symptoms. This is not because of any danger from excessive use of your reliever, but because needing Ventolin Evohaler or any other reliever drug every day is a warning sign that you need more preventive treatment to keep your asthma under better control.

A recent report from the Committee on Safety of Medicines looked very carefully at the use of relievers such as Ventolin Evohaler, and concluded that these drugs are quite safe when used as prescribed.

If Ventolin (or Bricanyl) is needed more frequently than every four hours or if the drug does not work within 15 minutes, this is an important danger sign and medical help is needed urgently. This very important point is dealt with in Chapter 6 on *Emergencies*.

Are any of these inhalers addictive?

No. Many people, particularly parents of children with asthma, worry that inhalers may be addictive. They fear that the more treatment you take, the more you will need. As a result they allow themselves, or their children, to suffer unpleasant symptoms that could have been avoided if the asthma treatment had been given. This concern is misplaced. Asthma drugs are not addictive, and you do not need to keep increasing the dose to get the same effect. If anything, the reverse is true, and asthma which is left untreated now may lead to larger amounts of drugs being required in the future, as well as to a permanent narrowing of the airways.

We all want to see maximum effect from the minimum treatment required, but sometimes it is necessary to take more treatment to get good control over the asthma. This is not because treatment is addictive, but because the asthma has become worse.

My daughter takes Intal four times daily. Is she becoming a 'drug addict' and if she stops taking the Intal will she have withdrawal symptoms?

No, she is certainly not becoming a drug addict! Intal is not in any way addictive. People can take it for many years and then can stop it abruptly without withdrawal symptoms – except perhaps a recurrence of their asthma. As we have seen in the section on *Drug treatments*, Intal is a very safe preventive treatment and the vast majority of people using it have no side effects. Occasionally, though, the powder in the spincaps can induce coughing which leads to wheezing.

I don't want to become dependent on my inhalers. Will this happen if I take them regularly?

The different types of inhalers fall into two categories – the relievers and the preventers (explained in more detail in the earlier section on *Drug treatments*). The reliever inhalers (e.g. Ventolin and Bricanyl) are generally best taken on an 'as required' basis rather than regularly. If they are taken regularly though, and by this we mean perhaps 4–6 times a day, it is possible to become reliant on them. This is not because the drug is addictive, but because they are probably being relied upon to give you relief from your asthma symptoms. Nowadays it is considered advisable to take preventive treatment if a reliever drug is needed more than once a day.

The preventer drugs (e.g. Becotide, Flixotide, Pulmicort, Intal and Tilade) do not give immediate relief and therefore you will not ever feel that you need to take them, so in this sense you will not become dependent on them. You may be required to take them regularly but this will be to keep your asthma well controlled. There is no doubt that your health, or even your life, may depend on taking the inhalers but you will not become addicted to them.

Aren't steroids harmful?

We should first make it clear that the steroids used in asthma treatment are not the same as the steroids abused by a few athletes. Those are *anabolic steroids*. In asthma we are concerned with a type called corticosteroids.

Corticosteroids now play a major role in the treatment of asthma. They are given in different ways – by the inhaled route, by mouth (*oral*) or by injection. Very low doses indeed are given by the inhaled route, and in standard doses almost none of the drug is absorbed into the body. Side effects in these circumstances are uncommon.

Steroid injections are not often given these days. They are nearly always reserved for acute attacks of asthma, particularly if someone is vomiting and unable to swallow tablets. On the other hand, steroid tablets are given very often for acute attacks. A short course of tablets, even in high doses, will have few side effects. Occasionally people notice some weight gain, or a mood change, but the effects are temporary. The advantages in taking a short course of steroids for an acute attack far outweigh the disadvantages. They can be life saving.

In people with severe asthma, taking steroid tablets long term, that is over months or years, can have serious side effects. These include weight gain, particularly a fullness of the face ('moon-face'), and a thinning of the skin leading to easy bruising. The blood pressure may increase, and there is a greater risk of developing diabetes in those prone to it. Other problems may be stomach ulceration and thinning of the bones. None of these problems is common, but all are recognized long-term risks with oral steroids. This is why, wherever possible, inhaled rather than oral steroids are given.

There is some concern that very high doses of the inhaled steroids may have some of the same effects over many years, but the evidence for normal dosages is very reassuring.

Are there any side effects from inhaled steroids?

When taken in **low** doses the only side effect of inhaled topical steroids is hoarseness of the voice. You can avoid this by using your inhaler before brushing your teeth, and by rinsing your mouth out very well. Thrush (otherwise known as monilia or candida infection) of the mouth may be a problem, more likely to occur at **higher** doses. In this case there is a red rash with white spots on the back of the throat which may irritate or cause voice problems. You can usually avoid this by using one of the large spacer inhaler devices (Volumatic [Figure 2.10], Nebuhaler [Figure 2.11], Aerochamber, Able Spacer, Integra and Babyhaler) and by eating some live natural yoghurt (which acts against the thrush) every day.

In very high doses there may be a small risk of thinning of the bones (osteoporosis). However, very high doses are only required when the alternatives are to have dangerously uncontrolled asthma, or to take steroid tablets long term.

Will the steroids stunt my child's growth?

We do not know in what form and in what dose your daughter is taking steroids. However, occasional short courses of oral steroids such as prednisolone will not affect your child's growth even when they are given in high doses. They are essential in the management of an acute asthma attack, and can be life saving. If these short courses are required several times each year, or if steroid tablets have to be taken over a long period of time – months or years – they can reduce growth in children.

The introduction of inhaled steroids in 1972 made a tremendous difference as far as this problem in children was concerned. It meant that asthma could be well controlled without the risks of long-term oral steroids. Despite this, there has still been concern that inhaled steroids might have an unfavourable effect on growth if given to children over a number of years. Much research has been carried out on the subject of growth following long-term inhaled steroid treatments. Contrary to expectations, growth actually improved in many children because the asthma was better controlled – asthma itself is often a cause of poor growth.

With higher doses (more than 800 micrograms per day) the picture is less clear. A balance must be drawn between the known effect of uncontrolled asthma in reducing children's growth, and the possible effect of high dose inhaled steroids in doing the same.

If your child is taking this sort of dose, discuss the problem with your doctor.

I am 72 years old, and have been told that my osteoporosis has probably got worse from being on Ventolin and Becotide for many years. How true is this?

Osteoporosis is gradual thinning and weakening of the bones due to a loss of calcium from the body. It occurs in all people to some extent as they become older. It results in an increased tendency to fractures, particularly of the hips and spine. Sometimes it is made worse as a side effect of steroid **tablets** but usually only after years of use. It is unlikely that your osteoporosis has become worse owing to your Becotide, unless you have been taking very high doses for several years or more. If you have, it is also likely that you will have required many short courses of steroid tablets for acute asthma, and the cumulative effect of these may have contributed. Ventolin does not have any effect whatsoever on osteoporosis.

It is worth bearing in mind that all women who have passed the menopause may develop osteoporosis. It occurs more often in smokers and those who do not take exercise. Hormone replacement therapy given during and after the menopause will help to retain the body's calcium stores and may prevent osteoporosis.

Why can't I always take prednisolone?

We have some sympathy with your question. Taking prednisolone (steroid) tablets on a regular basis and so keeping your asthma well controlled all the time seems, on the face of it, to be a very attractive suggestion. Some people see it as a way of dispensing with the regular use of inhalers. So why don't we recommend long term use of prednisolone, unless it is absolutely essential? The reason is because of important side effects.

Taking prednisolone **continuously** means that the level of steroid in the blood is always high. Because of this the *adrenal gland* makes less *cortisol*, which is the body's natural equivalent to prednisolone. Eventually after **long-term** use (**not** short-term) the adrenal gland becomes inactive. It stops producing cortisol itself, and the body comes to rely completely on the steroid tablets. Cortisol is produced by the body to cope with all kinds of stress, for example a serious illness. If the steroid tablets are, for some reason, stopped suddenly the adrenal gland cannot make up the difference. In this case, the body is dangerously prone to illness. This explains why people taking long-term steroid treatment need to carry warning cards to show to any doctor treating them.

There are other serious side effects that can occur if prednisolone is taken over many years. These include skin changes, thinning of the bones, increases in blood pressure, indigestion and ulcers, and development of diabetes. This is an alarming list, and we must emphasize that these risks are **not** present with the use of **short** courses of prednisolone which we favour for treating uncontrolled and acute asthma, unless a large number of such courses are required over a number of years.

A small minority of people with chronic severe asthma do find that inhaled steroids, even in high doses, are not sufficient to control symptoms. In these cases doctors have little choice but to prescribe regular doses of steroid tablets. Side effects are much more likely to occur in these cases if the dose needed is above 5 milligrams per day taken over a long period of time.

Why do I keep getting white spots on the back of my throat?

It is likely that you have thrush infection in your throat. This is also known as *candida* or *monilia infection*, but is best known as 'thrush'. It is a fungus infection, and is one of the very few side effects caused by inhaled steroids. Fortunately thrush can be treated effectively using an antifungal treatment in liquid or lozenge form.

The chances of it recurring can be reduced in several ways. The simplest is to rinse out your mouth and clean your teeth whenever you use your preventer inhaler. Another way, particularly when higher doses are prescribed, is to use a spacer device (Aerochamber, Volumatic, Nebuhaler or Integra – Figures 2.10, 2.11). These chambers allow the larger particles of the drug (which are the likely cause of thrush) to be held in the chamber rather than be deposited in the mouth and throat.

Does any of my asthma medication affect my immune system?

This depends on what treatment you are taking and in what dose. Very few people with asthma have to take so much treatment that their immune system is affected, but it is possible. Steroid tablets (prednisolone) taken over a long period of time can affect the immune system. The result of this is that someone may suffer more infections than normal, or may not be able to fight infections as effectively as other people. One way of reducing the risk of prednisolone side effects is to take the tablets on alternate days rather than every day. There are no effects on the immune system if you only need to take occasional short courses of steroid tablets each year.

In theory at least, inhaled topical steroids in very high doses may also pose a risk of affecting the immune system, although there is little or no evidence to confirm this. High doses are generally agreed to be above 800 micrograms daily of Becotide (beclomethasone dipropionate) or Pulmicort (budesonide) and 400 micrograms of Flixotide in children, and twice this in adults. Fortunately not many people need such high doses. In those who do, one way of reducing side effects is to use a large spacer device (Nebuhaler for Pulmicort; Volumatic for Becotide or Flixotide).

I read in the paper that asthma treatments are dangerous. Is this true?

Asthma itself is dangerous. Any dangers of drug treatments need to be carefully balanced against the dangers of asthma. In low doses there are no serious side effects for any of the asthma medications. As the doses are increased, then the risks of side effects are greater. However, doses are only increased when a person's asthma is worse, and therefore they are at more risk.

High doses of steroids over long periods of time, whether in the form of tablets or by the inhaled route, may cause side effects. The most serious of these are thinning of the bones (osteoporosis) and a reduced ability to fight infections. These risks can be reduced by using one of the large spacer devices (Nebuhaler, Volumatic,

Aerochamber or Able Spacer) if taking a high dose of inhaled topical steroid (eg Becloforte or Pulmicort 200).

The theophylline drugs (aminophylline, Nuelin, Slo-Phyllin, Uniphyllin) may be dangerous if their levels in the blood are too high. Anyone taking these drugs should have a blood test from time to time to check that the levels are satisfactory. Some other drugs increase the risk of problems with theophyllines. These include erythromycin (an antibiotic), and cimetidine (Tagamet – an anti-ulcer drug). Always check with your doctor if you are prescribed these drugs.

Generally our aim is for you to control your asthma with the lowest possible dose of a drug. This is achieved best if the effects of your asthma are regularly reviewed. This is covered in Chapter 3.

I have a young child who has asthma. What are the effects and side effects of Ventolin syrup?

Ventolin syrup is a reliever drug which, as its name implies, is swallowed rather than inhaled. The active drug is exactly the same as Ventolin (generic name salbutamol) taken in nebulizers or inhalers. However, it needs to be taken in a higher dose than inhaled Ventolin, because it has to be taken up into the blood stream and circulated all round the body before reaching the lungs. Inhaled Ventolin goes straight to the lungs and not into the bloodstream. The side effects of Ventolin syrup are shaking (or trembling) of the hands, and pounding (or racing) of the heart. These are the same side effects that some people feel when they take a lot of Ventolin through their inhaler. A few children may become hyperactive when taking Ventolin syrup. This is unusual, and happens much less often than with other drugs. It always disappears if the medicine is stopped.

Will steroids affect my daughter's potential growth?

They could do, but it depends on how she takes them, what dose she takes and for how long. It's important to look at different aspects of treating asthma with steroids, and to take them one by one. Firstly, if steroid tablets are given for a prolonged length of time (months or longer) to children, they certainly do slow down growth. There are very few children who require steroid tablets to this extent. In those that do, growth is less likely to be affected if the steroid tablets can be taken on alternate days.

Secondly, we are now in the fortunate position of being able to use low dose **inhaled** steroids as preventive agents. These are extremely effective, and at usual doses it is known that they will not have any effect on a child's growth. Care must to be taken when higher doses are needed to control the asthma. When inhaled steroid dosages are increased on a long-term basis it is important to weigh up all considerations. We should always aim to give minimal treatment for maximum effect. If the higher doses of inhaled steroids are needed, then the use of spacer devices will reduce the risk of side effects, including the slowing down of growth. It is important to monitor every child's growth during the course of their asthma treatment.

Thirdly, it should be remembered that uncontrolled chronic asthma can itself cause slowing down of growth. In fact, the introduction of inhaled steroids often promotes growth because the asthma improves.

Finally, it is interesting that many children with asthma have a delayed puberty, and their adolescent growth spurt is held up. Once puberty and the growth spurt do occur, the eventual height reached is at least that predicted from their earlier growth performance, and can be above average.

Does inhaled Ventolin Evohaler affect tooth enamel?

Using Ventolin Evohaler in an aerosol inhaler should not affect your teeth. Dry powder capsules do contain lactose, which is a type of sugar, but this should not add significantly to tooth decay. Tooth enamel is damaged by sugar because the sugar ferments in your mouth and produces acid, and the acid then attacks the enamel. However, the amount of lactose contained in a dry powder capsule is very small, and in any case lactose tends to be less harmful than the sugars we put into tea or coffee, or which we eat in sweets and biscuits.

You can also further reduce any risk to your teeth by cleaning them after using your inhaler. This may be difficult in the middle of the day, but is perfectly easy to fit into your night and morning routine.

Can inhaled steroids ever make children hyperactive and cause sleep problems?

Not that we are aware of, but in medicine even the most unlikely things **can** happen!

Steroid tablets taken in high doses can occasionally cause side effects such as mood changes, nightmares and mental disturbances. However, it is very rare indeed for inhaled steroids to have any sort of effect on the central nervous system. A few cases of unusual mood changes have been reported to the Committee of Safety of Medicines by the doctors of patients taking beclomethasone dipropionate (Beconase, Becotide or Becloforte). It is important to realize, though, that the reporting of such an event to the Committee does not necessarily mean that it has been caused by the drug. The events may have occurred for other reasons in the people taking the medication.

We should re-emphasize that the incidence of serious side effects for people using inhaled steroids is very low. This risk must be compared with the relief obtained from their use without any untoward effects.

I have heard that CFCs are due to be phased out – what will happen to asthma inhalers?

You are quite right. In order to protect the Earth's atmosphere, the substances (*propellants*) that provide the energy for the pressurized asthma inhalers (the CFCs – which stands for chlorofluorocarbons) are to be phased out completely in the near future. Fortunately the pharmaceutical companies have collaborated and developed two new substances – HFA-134a and HFA-227 (hydrofluoroalkane propellants). These will be used as energy sources for future inhalers. As soon as two HFA (CFC-free) inhalers have been produced for a particular drug, no new licences will be issued for the CFC products. For example, as soon as two CFC-free inhalers containing beclomethasone are licensed in a country, the authorities will no longer allow pharmaceutical companies to produce CFC-containing beclomethasone inhalers.

In the UK these include Aerobec, Becotide, Becloforte, Beclazone and Filair.

Two HFA (CFC-free) pressurized inhalers have been licensed for use in the United Kingdom. These are Airomir (salbutamol) a reliever, and Qvar (beclomethasone) a preventer; both manufactured by 3M Pharmaceuticals. Doctors have been advised to prescribe Qvar by this name (the trade name) rather than as a 'generic' prescription (i.e. beclomethasone) and at half the dose of the CFC beclomethasone products. The reason for this is that Qvar achieves the same effect at half the dose as the CFC beclomethasone preparations (Aerobec, Asmabec, Becotide, Becloforte, Beclazone and Filair).

3
Monitoring and Control

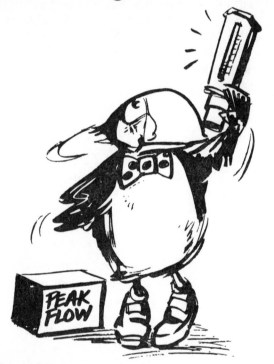

Introduction

Success in looking after your asthma hinges on knowing how and when to make adjustments in your treatment in response to changes in your condition. Getting the treatment right in the first place is a partnership between you and your doctor, asthma nurse and other health professionals. Once you have your treatment, you are the person who has to live with your asthma and identify when your symptoms change. From our viewpoint, the best way to do this is to use a combination of symptoms and peak expiratory flow readings (assuming you are able to use a peak flow meter). Peak flow meters are available on prescription on the NHS. Individual peak flow meters do give different results, therefore it is best to have your own meter. There are many people who do have meters, but take their readings only occasionally. This can be fine, as long as you appreciate that symptoms usually start some time after peak expiratory flow readings have started to fall.

There are approximately 100 000 hospital admissions for acute asthma every year in the UK. Many of these attacks could be avoided by prompt action, as long as the attack is recognized early. We believe that helping you to recognize *uncontrolled asthma* is one of the most important functions of this book. Uncontrolled asthma means **danger** and we urge you to read this section carefully. One of the biggest changes in asthma care in recent years has been the advent of asthma clinics in general practice, to complement the asthma clinics in hospitals. The first section deals with these types of clinic, and the roles of doctors and asthma nurses. Some asthma clinics are much more established than others, so there will be a good deal of variation in the way that they run. Much effort is being put into improving the all round organization and levels of care that we can offer in this way to people with asthma.

Seeing the doctor – and asthma clinics

Do I need to see my GP every time I think asthma is coming, or just use my inhaler?

The answer to this question is rather complex, because it is dependent on a number of factors, of which two are perhaps the most important: firstly the severity of your asthma, and secondly the type of inhaled treatment you use.

Ideally, you should agree a self-management plan with your doctor or asthma nurse. This plan will deal with what should happen when your asthma symptoms get worse, and usually there will be one or more steps that you can take before seeking help.

This may be one simple step, such as increasing the dose of reliever inhaler. On the other hand, it may be a number of steps, up to and including starting a course of steroid tablets before seeing your doctor.

This plan can be reviewed with your doctor or at an asthma clinic after an attack of asthma, when it may be necessary to change some steps in treatment to try and prevent another attack.

There is a section on *Self-management plans* further on in this chapter.

How often should I see my doctor or go to the clinic?

This varies greatly, depending on the type and severity of your asthma. Some people only suffer from asthma during certain times of the year, for example the hay fever season. In these cases, it may be necessary to be reviewed only once a year. On the other hand, people who have very severe asthma may need to attend the surgery or clinic every month or so.

There are some special times when it is particularly important to see the doctor or asthma nurse for review of your asthma.

● Everyone should be reviewed soon after an attack of asthma severe enough to need a dose of emergency nebulized bronchodilator. Regardless of whether such treatment took place in the surgery, at home or in hospital, an appointment should be booked as soon as possible. It is always difficult to predict how long an attack will take to clear up completely, but a daily peak flow chart will help. The clinic is an ideal place to review this chart and decide how to continue the treatment. Those involved can also try to work out why the attack occurred and decide what needs to be done in order to prevent another.

● A clinic appointment for review before going on holiday is helpful. Self-management plans are often needed when on holiday and may even save lives. Spare inhaler prescriptions are a good idea as well.

My doctor says I would benefit from attending his asthma clinic. What is this and what happens there?

General practitioners frequently provide a range of clinics where particular conditions (such as asthma or diabetes) or particular problems (such as stopping smoking or preventing heart disease) are dealt with in one clinic rather than in the usual mixed surgeries. Some of these clinics are run by the GP, whilst others are run by the practice nurse. In some cases both the GP and the nurse run the clinic together. The main advantage of such clinics for asthma is that they usually provide more time to talk. There are many things to learn about asthma and these can't easily be dealt with in a busy surgery with five or 10 minute appointments. The clinic setting allows more time to deal with questions, particularly for those people whose asthma has recently been diagnosed. This book is an attempt to answer many of the questions which crop up repeatedly, but it is also helpful to talk to someone who is experienced in dealing with asthma.

A major problem in asthma care arises from the difficulties in arranging regular follow-up and monitoring of people with asthma. These may occur because:

- the GP doesn't seem to have the time;
- the GP doesn't think follow-up is needed;
- the GP doesn't offer follow-up appointments;
- the person with asthma doesn't take up the offer of an appointment;
- the person with asthma feels well and fails to keep the appointment.

A GP's asthma clinic surgery offers some solutions to these problems. It is often more convenient and less crowded than a hospital clinic. The practice asthma nurse can check that the people on the practice asthma register are offered regular appointments to be seen, and she can make contact with people who do not attend.

If you are on a practice's asthma register, how many people (such as future employers) have access to this information?

Nobody should have access to this information without your

express permission. An *asthma register* is a document or computer file held by a practice in order to help organize its asthma care. It is confidential to the practice.

Your own medical record held by your GP is also strictly confidential. Information about your health cannot be given to anyone – by your GP or any of the practice staff – without your written consent. In addition, you have the right to see that information before it is forwarded to an employer, an insurance company or anybody else, as long as you arrange to do so within 21 days of the request. If you are unwilling for the contents to be forwarded, you can ask for them to be withheld, although your GP will have to disclose that you have made this request.

Always ask to discuss this issue with your GP if you are concerned about other people having access to your medical details. Confidentiality is one of the most important parts of the relationship between health professionals and patients.

Why do I need to come to a clinic?

There are many important aspects to asthma and its treatment. An asthma clinic in general practice should offer more time than the usual surgery appointments, and should be run by someone with a special interest in asthma. This extra time and experience offers obvious benefits to you and your family. Many hospitals also run asthma clinics now in preference to general chest clinics, and these have specially trained staff who can assist people with asthma in their understanding and management of the condition.

Of course clinics vary from practice to practice and between hospitals. Generally, though, they will concentrate on the following things:

- making sure that the inhaler device that has been prescribed is suitable;
- checking to make sure that the inhaler is being used effectively;
- answering questions and discussing concerns people may have about asthma;
- helping people recognize when their asthma is going out of control, and how to deal with emergencies;
- teaching about the use of peak expiratory flow readings;

- helping people understand more about their asthma and the medication used;
- helping people to prevent attacks by using their improved understanding of treatments and peak flow meters.

An asthma clinic should offer you the best possible opportunity for discussing **your** asthma and any concerns you may have about your treatment or progress.

I have had repeat prescriptions for several years now, and haven't seen my doctor. What shall I do?

We advise you very strongly to see your doctor. If your practice runs an asthma clinic, then ask to attend. If not, see your doctor in surgery time. If your doctor does not seem interested in asthma, and you are worried by your symptoms, ask to be referred to a specialist at your local hospital. Asthma treatment policy changes from time to time, and your treatment should be reviewed, and may need to be changed. Inhalers are not easy to use correctly so it is worth having your technique checked. It may be better to switch to a different device if your technique turns out to be faulty.

It may be that your asthma is mild, or just that you manage it very effectively by yourself, but it is always nice for the doctor and nurse to see someone who is controlling their asthma successfully!

Can my husband be referred for tests to see what's causing it?

There are no definitive tests to see what causes asthma. There are allergy tests, but often these are not very helpful. The most common type is called a skin prick test, in which various substances, or allergens, are pricked into the skin. If the skin reacts and swells up, then the person is probably allergic to that substance. The difficulty is that allergy in the skin is not necessarily the same as allergy in the nose or lungs. Nine times out of ten, a person will know already to which substances they are allergic, because they sneeze or wheeze on direct contact. Allergy tests often serve only to confirm a fact already known to the sufferer. However, these investigations may help to identify new trigger factors.

Special tests can measure the amount of antibodies (substances produced by the body's immune system) to certain allergens in the blood. If someone has an allergy which is important in causing symptoms, then the levels of antibodies in the blood are very high. The tests are expensive and complicated to interpret. In a few cases they are very important, but in most they are unhelpful in dealing with the asthma.

Known triggers of asthma should be avoided by sufferers if at all possible. These will usually be known to the person or family.

What is the role of the doctor in controlling asthma?

The doctor probably has the most important role in diagnosis of asthma and in beginning the right treatment. After this, however, other people become more important in the day-to-day control of the condition. Most important of all is the person with asthma – you! You are the one who has to take the treatment day in and day out, to recognize symptoms of asthma coming on, and to take action to deal with them. Contact with doctors forms only a tiny proportion of day-to-day living. This is why it is essential for people with asthma to take an active part in the control of their own condition, so that they are able to lead their lives as fully as possible, unrestricted by their asthma.

Increasingly, nurses with special training in asthma care are playing a major part in providing them with the knowledge and skills to do this. These nurses work in hospital asthma clinics, in general practice and in schools.

Having said all this, the doctor does retain vital roles in the ongoing management of asthma. These are:

- to prescribe suitable medication;
- to follow up people with asthma when they are well;
- to help people with asthma and their families to monitor their asthma, and to recognize when asthma is going out of control;
- to treat in cases of emergency.

What is the role of a practice nurse in the prevention and treatment of asthma?

This depends a great deal on the practice and the individual nurse concerned. Many general practices are now devoting much more time to looking after people with asthma, and the practice nurse can play a major role. Since April 1990, when major changes were made in GPs' terms of service, many have been running asthma clinics in their practices. Often there is a system of shared care between the GP and the nurse and in this the nurse may play a fairly minimal role – perhaps recording the patient's peak flow measurements and demonstrating inhaler technique – whilst the GP carries out all the other aspects of management. In many practices nurses are now extending their role successfully, to include:

- obtaining a full asthma history;
- recording and interpreting peak expiratory flow readings;
- confirming the diagnosis of asthma;
- constructing appropriate anticipatory/preventive asthma treatment plans in partnership with the person with asthma and the GP;
- demonstrating, teaching and checking inhaler technique;
- providing relevant education and counselling to enable someone to carry out 'guided' self-management;
- setting up a well organized, regular system for review of symptoms, lung function, treatment and delivery systems;
- being readily accessible to give advice.

We do not believe that nurses should be asked to take on this degree of responsibility without receiving specialized training. Many practice nurses have now done this, and developed a high level of expertise. Their objectives are to help people maintain optimum control of their own asthma, and to minimize its effect on their lives.

It is important that at least one GP in the practice is also particularly interested and knowledgeable about asthma. There is no doubt that people with asthma will receive the most effective care if there is teamwork and good co-operation of the GP, the nurse and the hospital.

How do I let my GP know what I want, when he seems to want to be in charge?

You have asked about one of the most important areas in the practice of medicine. Good communication between GPs and their patients is absolutely vital if the best outcome for any long-term problem is to be achieved. Sadly, poor communication occurs far more often than we would like. GPs often fail to understand what patients' needs are. People often fail to under-stand why GPs are worried about them, and how they are trying to treat their asthma (or other problems).

In an ideal situation your GP or nurse will take care to find out what you expect from the consultation. In asthma, you should be given an opportunity to show how much you know about your asthma, and your feelings about treatment. The GP or nurse can then explain the facts and discuss treatment choices with you in a meaningful way. Following this you can both agree on a treatment plan. Unfortunately this does not always happen!

People's expectations are very different. Some visit the GP hoping for a prescription which will cure their problem. Others wish to discuss their health, and then make their own decision on treatment. The GP–patient relationship should be a two-sided one, with both having a say in the treatment plan. Friction usually results from a failure on both sides to communicate clearly. In your own case it may be difficult because your GP believes that he knows what is the best treatment. He may feel defensive if you have another viewpoint which challenges his own. For example, you may be seeking a cure for asthma while your GP may believe the best course of action is to avoid attacks by taking regular preventive treatment. In your own case think carefully about the points you wish to discuss before you go in to see your GP. Try not to leave before you have discussed them! It may help to take your partner or a friend along with you.

Sometimes GPs and patients cannot get along with each other no matter how hard they try. When this happens it may be best to agree to differ, and to change to another doctor.

Peak expiratory flow monitoring

Why do I need to use a peak flow meter?

Because it gives you a lot of information about your asthma!

The peak flow meter (Figure 3.1) gives a reading (peak expiratory flow or PEF) which tells how open your airways are. The more widely open the airways, the higher the rate at which air can be blown out of the lungs, and the higher the reading. Normal PEF readings may be anywhere between 400 and 550 *litres per minute* for adult women, and 500 and 650 for men. During episodes of asthma, the airways become narrowed, and the PEF falls.

So measuring the PEF can help to show you when an attack is on the way. Often it will show a drop in readings a few days before symptoms develop. In this way it helps you to decide when to increase your medication to prevent an attack or episode of uncontrolled asthma.

In a different way, the PEF can be of help in confirming that your asthma control is good. If your PEF readings are regularly around your best readings, and there is not very much variation, then your asthma is well controlled. In other words your PEFs are almost the same every day and night, and at or close to your best reading. We prefer to take the best value achieved by someone whenever possible, since 'normal values' are based on sex, age and height, and have a wide range.

At what times of day should I record my peak expiratory flow?

Some people take their PEF religiously, before and after treat-

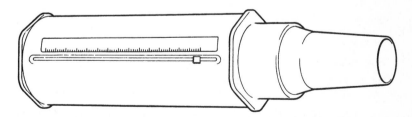

Figure 3.1   The Clement Clarke Standard Range Peak Flow Meter, which is one of the various types of peak flow meter available.

ment, several times daily. Most, however, find this totally impractical and find it difficult to keep up peak flow diaries on a daily basis. We appreciate how difficult it is to maintain this routine, month after month, particularly when your asthma is under good control. From our point of view, recording your PEF twice daily, before any reliever treatment, is perfectly adequate to give a good record of your asthma. The best times to take these readings are in the morning soon after waking, in the afternoon, and at night before going to bed. Make a note of the best of three blows whenever you take your PEF. Morning readings alone are helpful, but it is really best to do afternoon and/or night readings as well, because this shows how your asthma varies from beginning to end of the day.

Your readings can be written down in simple number form such as in Figure 3.2. The chart shows that the PEF readings are sometimes very low and at times a lot higher. It is not difficult to see that these readings show that the person's asthma is out of control. There are two things that show this.

Day	Morning Readings (Best of 3)	Evening Readings (Best of 3)
Monday 25th	230	200
Tuesday 26th	300	350
Wednesday 27th	300	330
Thursday 28th	350	350
Friday 29th	330	370
Saturday 30th	320	400
Sunday 31st	350	320
Monday 1st	250	250
Tuesday 2nd	300	290
Wednesday 3rd	250	340
Thursday 4th	280	250

Figure 3.2 A peak flow record showing a child's readings. They are very different from morning to night and from day to day; therefore this child has severely uncontrolled asthma.

- Look at the highest and the lowest readings. In this chart the lowest is 200 and the highest is 400, so the readings are very different, as the highest is double the lowest. When asthma is well controlled, there should be very little difference between the day to day readings or between the morning and evening readings.
- Look at the difference between the morning and the evening readings on the same days. In this chart the morning and the evening readings are sometimes almost the same and at other times very different. This gives an idea of the variation from morning to evening – called the diurnal variation.

Like many other people, you may find that graphs are a lot easier to follow. The peak flow chart in Figure 3.3 shows the same child's PEF readings as shown in number form in Figure 3.2. There are a few things to look for in peak flow graphs.

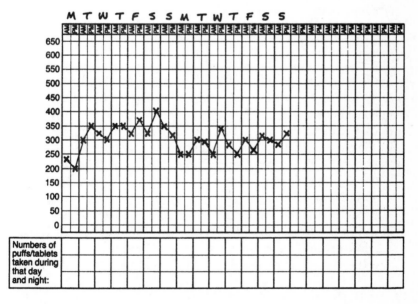

Figure 3.3   This graph shows peak flow readings from a child whose asthma is out of control.

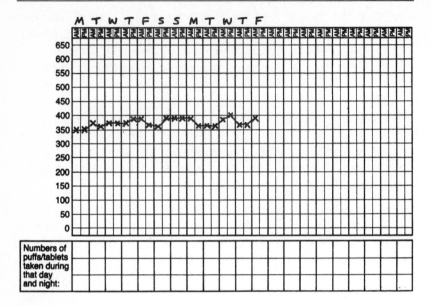

Figure 3.4   This is a peak flow chart showing well controlled asthma. The readings are almost level with little change from day to day or from morning to evening.

- Look at the pattern. Normal peak flow graphs should be almost level (as in Figure 3.4). The graph in Figure 3.3 shows very uneven lines.
- Look at the gap between the morning and the evening readings. In Figure 3.3, on the first Monday they go from 230 to 200. On the next day, Tuesday, they go from 300 to 350. The difference between these readings is too great, indicating that the child's asthma is out of control.
- Look at the change from day to day. This is easier to see on the graph in Figure 3.3 than the chart with the numbers in Figure 3.2. For example, the change from the Monday to the Tuesday, and the change from the Sunday to the Monday is very clear.

How useful can a peak flow meter be?

Very useful, as it gives a measurement that shows how tight your airways are. When your asthma is well controlled, your twice daily

LIST OF PLATES

Plate 1 DRUG AND TRADEMARK TABLES

Table A: Generic and brand names of drugs

Asthma drugs	Generic name	Brand names
Reliever inhalers – short-acting	salbutamol	Aerolin, Asmasal Clickhaler, Airomir, Salamol, Salbulin, Ventolin, Ventolin Evohaler
	terbutaline	Bricanyl
Reliever inhalers – longer acting	salmeterol xinofoate	Serevent
	eformoterol fumarate	Foradil, Oxis
Reliever tablets	aminophylline	Phyllocontin
	bambuterol	Bambec
	orciprenaline	Alupent
	salbutamol	Volmax
	terbutaline	Bricanyl
	theophylline	Nuelin, Uniphyllin
Preventer inhalers	beclomethasone dipropionate	Aerobec, Asmabec Clickhaler, Becloforte, Beclazone, Becotide, Filair, Qvar
	budesonide	Pulmicort
	fluticasone propionate	Flixotide
	nedocromil sodium	Tilade
	sodium cromoglycate	Intal, Cromogen
Leukotriene receptor antagonist tablets	montelukast sodium	Singulair
	zafirlukast	Accolate
Combinations	salmeterol xinafolate + fluticasone propionate	Seretide (Serevent + Flixotide)
	beclomethasone dipropionate + salbutamol	Ventide

Table B: Trademarks

Manufacturer	Drugs	Devices	Spacers
Allen & Hanburys (A member of the GlaxoWellcome group of companies)	Becloforte, Serevent Becotide, Ventolin Flixotide, Seretide, Ventide	pMDI (not Seretide), Accuhaler (not Becotide/ Becloforte) Diskhaler Rotahaler (Ventolin, Becotide only) Easi-Breathe (Ventolin, Becotide/Becloforte) Evohaler (Ventolin)	Babyhaler Integra (Becloforte only) Volumatic
AstraZeneca	Accolate tablets Pulmicort, Bricanyl Oxis	pMDI (not Oxis), Turbohaler	Nebuhaler
Aventis	Aerocrom Intal Tilade	pMDI Spinhaler Syncroner	Fisonair
Celltech Medeva	Asmasal Asmabec	Clickhaler	
Clement Clarke International Ltd		In-Check, In-Check Dial Mini-Wright peak flow meter Windmill Trainer	Able Spacer
MSD	Singulair tablets		
Norton Healthcare	Beclazone, Salamol Cromogen	Easi-Breathe	
Novartis	Foradil	Breath-actuated inhaler	
3M Health Care	Aerobec, Airomir, Aerolin, Filair, Nuelin, Qvar, Salbulin	Autohaler, pMDI	Aerochamber

CFC-free pMDI inhalers: Ventolin Evohaler: Allen & Hanburys; Airomir, Qvar, Salbulin: 3M
The names of the products listed above are trademarks of the manufacturers.

Plate 2   DISKHALER

The Diskhaler by Allen & Hanburys is designed for use with Ventolin (salbutamol), which is a short-acting reliever. There are other versions of this device, designed for use with other asthma medications. Serevent (salmeterol – a long-acting reliever) Diskhalers are coloured green; Becotide and Becloforte (beclomethasone dipropionate – a preventer) Diskhalers are coloured brown or maroon, and Flixotide (fluticasone propionate – a preventer) Diskhalers are coloured orange. Remember, you should always discuss the use of your device with your doctor or asthma nurse.

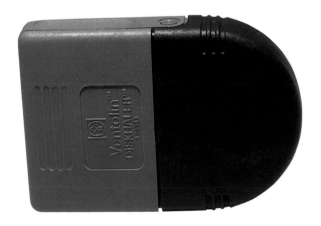

Plate 3 ACCUHALER

The Accuhaler by Allen & Hanburys contains Seretide (salmeterol/fluticasone), which is a combination of a long-acting reliever and a corticosteroid. It has a dose counter allowing you to monitor the number of doses taken. The device is also available containing Serevent (salmeterol), a long-acting reliever (coloured green), Flixotide (fluticasone propionate), a corticosteroid (coloured orange) and Ventolin (salbutamol), a short-acting reliever (coloured blue). Remember, you should always discuss the use of your device with your doctor or asthma nurse.

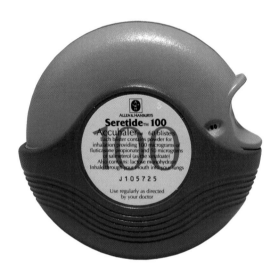

Plate 4 AUTOHALER

The Autohaler is a breath-actuated device by 3M that contains either the reliever medicine Airomir (CFC-free salbutamol), in which case the top of the Autohaler is coloured blue, or the preventer medicine Qvar (CFC-free beclomethasone), in which case the top of the Autohaler is coloured maroon or beige, depending on the medicine's strength. Remember to always discuss the use of your device with your doctor or asthma nurse.

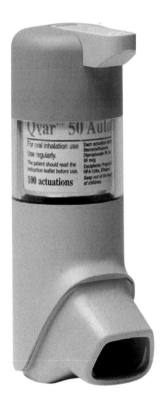
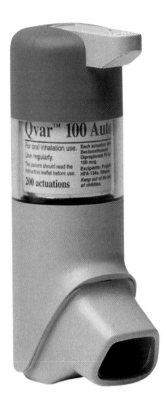

Plate 5   METERED DOSE INHALER (MDI) (3M)

Most asthma treatments are available in metered dose inhalers, and although the shape may differ slightly from one manufacturer to another (this one is from 3M), all manufacturers in the UK use the same colours to indicate what type of medicine is contained:

- blue is for relievers
- brown, beige, maroon or orange (depending on strength) are for preventers
- white with a red cap is for Intal
- yellow with a green cap is for Tilade
- green is for Serevent.

Be especially careful with inhalers that have been imported from overseas. They might not follow this colour system. Always discuss the use of your device with your doctor or asthma nurse.

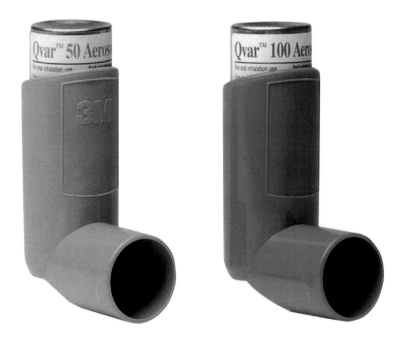

Plate 6   EASI-BREATHE

Easi-Breathe is a breath-actuated metered dose inhaler. Allen & Hanburys' products available for use in this device are Ventolin (salbutamol), a short-acting reliever, and Becotide and Becloforte (beclomethasone dipropionate), which are preventers. It is designed to remove the need for coordinating activation and inspiration, as the device actuates when you inhale. Remember, you should always discuss the use of your device with your doctor or asthma nurse.

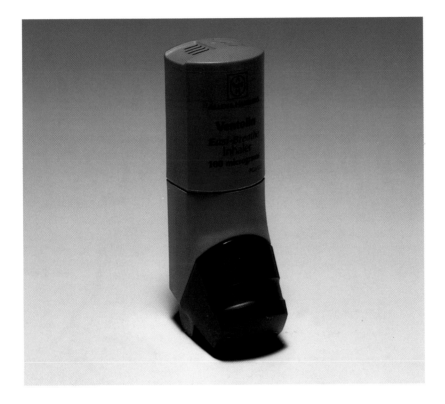

Plate 7 VENTOLIN EVOHALER

The Ventolin Evohaler is a CFC-free metered dose inhaler produced by Allen & Hanburys. Ventolin (salbutamol), a short-acting reliever, is available in this inhaler. The Ventolin Evohaler replaces the CFC-containing Ventolin inhaler. Remember, you should always discuss the use of your device with your doctor or asthma nurse.

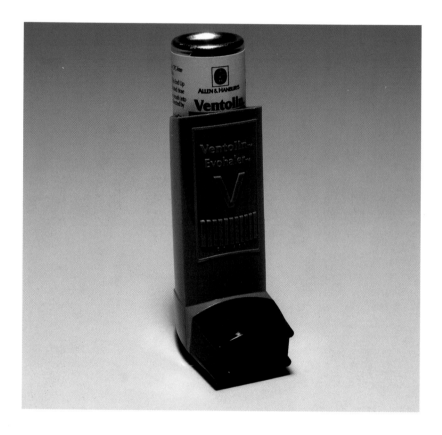

Plate 8   METERED DOSE INHALER (MDI) (A&H)

This device is a metered dose inhaler, and most asthma treatments are available in this form. This one is from Allen & Hanburys. The usual colours are:

- blue for relievers
- brown, maroon or orange for preventers (inhaled steroids)
- white with a red cap for Intal
- yellow with a green cap for Tilade
- green for Serevent (salmeterol).

All MDIs made by the manufacturers in this book are coloured in this way. However, the colours may be different, for example on those devices imported from abroad. Remember, you should always discuss the use of your device with your doctor or asthma nurse.

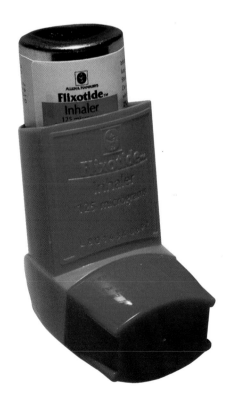

Plate 9   CLICKHALER

The Clickhaler by Celltech Medeva is a CFC-free, lactose carrier dry powder inhaler. It contains 200 doses (the Asmabec Clickhaler 250 µg contains 100 doses). There is a dose counter and a red indicator for the last 10 doses. The device locks when empty. Remember, you should always discuss the use of your device with your doctor or asthma nurse.

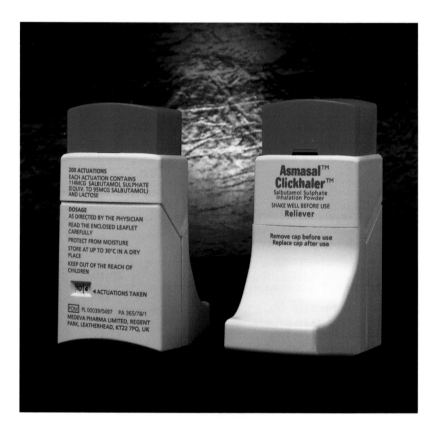

Plate 10   IN-CHECK DIAL

The In-Check Dial by Clement Clarke is a training tool to help teach the correct technique for different inhalers. Some inhalers need a fast inhalation, others only work best when you inhale through them slowly. This device can simulate different inhalers, and then measure the speed of air that you can breathe in. Remember, you should always discuss the use of your device with your doctor or asthma nurse.

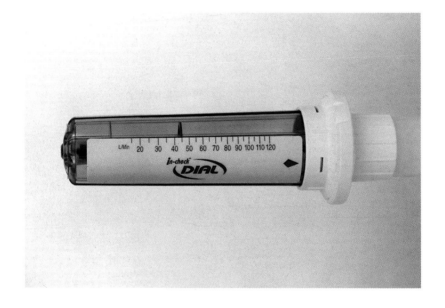

Plate 11   AEROCHAMBER

The AeroChamber by 3M is a compact and portable low-volume spacer device. It can be used with any asthma metered dose inhaler. The adult version is shown here and is available with either a mask or a mouth-piece. There is another version of the AeroChamber designed especially for children, and one for babies and infants. Remember to always discuss the use of your device with your doctor or asthma nurse.

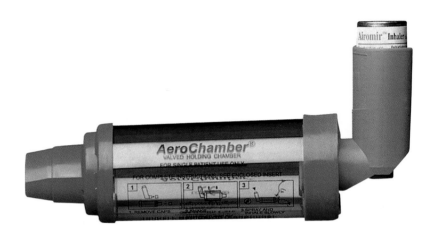

Plate 12   VOLUMATIC

The Volumatic by Allen & Hanburys is a large volume spacer device. There are two versions of this device, one designed for use by adults and older children, and a young paediatric version with a mask designed for giving treatment to babies and young children. Both versions can be used with any of the asthma metered dose inhalers made by Allen & Hanburys. Remember, you should always discuss the use of your device with your doctor or asthma nurse.

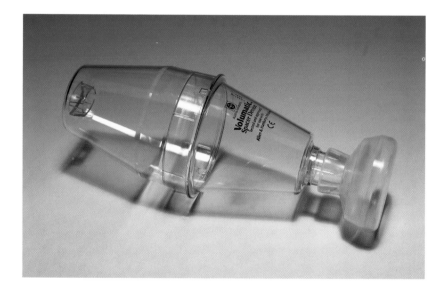

Plate 13   BABYHALER

The Babyhaler by Allen & Hanburys is a spacer device with a mask designed for giving treatment to babies and young children. It can be used with either Ventolin (salbutamol), which is a reliever, Becotide (beclomethasone) or Flixotide (fluticasone), which are preventers. Remember, you should always discuss the use of your device with your doctor or asthma nurse.

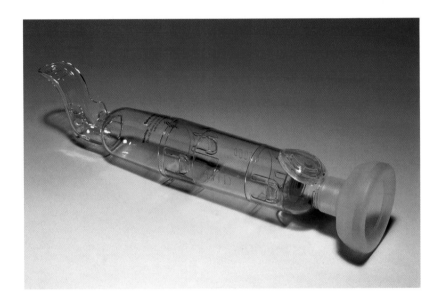

Plate 14 ABLE SPACER

The Able Spacer is made by Clement Clarke and can be used with all the commonly used pressurized metered dose inhaler (MDI) devices. This small volume spacer can store the MDI inside it, making it suitable for the active person with asthma. To improve inhaler technique, the Able Spacer 'whistles' if you inhale too quickly. A mask can be fitted to the mouthpiece, if recommended by your doctor or nurse. Remember, you should always discuss the use of your device with your doctor or asthma nurse.

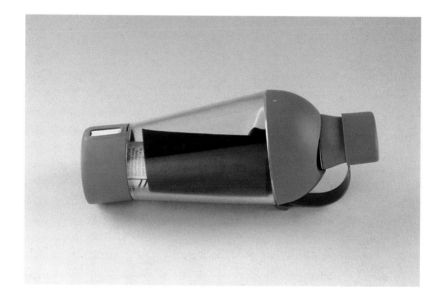

Plate 15 PEAK FLOW METER

A: This is the Clement Clarke Mini-Wright Peak Flow Meter, one of the various peak flow meters available. They are available in two versions:

Standard Range (60–800 l/min) has a black scale;
AFS Low Range (30–400 l/min) has a red scale.

Those with lower peak flows (children and the elderly) are best suited to the AFS Low Range, whilst older children (9–10 years and above) and adults normally use the Standard Range meter.

A

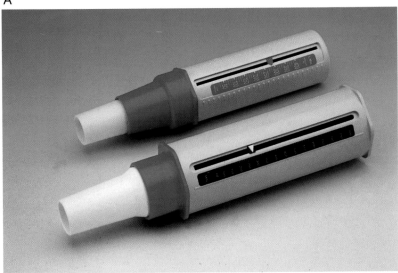

B: The Windmill Trainer has been attached to this boy's peak flow meter – by moving it further up the scale, more and more effort is needed to make the sails of the windmill turn. This helps to teach good peak flow technique and provide motivation for the younger asthmatic.

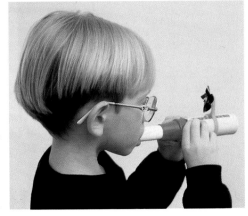

B

readings should be almost the same every time they are taken, although the evening reading is usually a little higher. They should not vary by more than about 15%. An example of a peak flow chart showing good asthma control is shown in Figure 3.4.

The main clue to uncontrolled asthma is irregular readings; in other words when the readings change a lot from day to day, trouble is on the way. Figures 3.2 and 3.3 show PEF readings of poorly controlled asthma.

The charts can be used in a number of ways but first you need to find out what your normal readings should be. Most doctors and nurses use the 'best ever' reading as the 'normal'. The best way to find out your normal or 'best ever' reading is to take some readings when your asthma is well controlled. Once you know your normal readings it becomes easy to see when your asthma is going (or has gone) out of control.

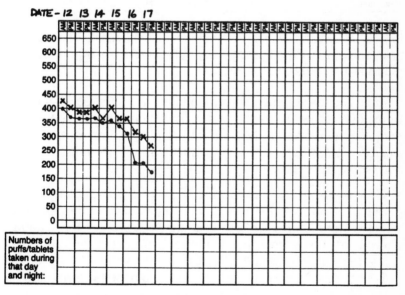

Figure 3.5 This chart shows an attack of asthma. The peak flow readings drop suddenly from 400 to 170 over 24 hours. Urgent relief medication and medical help are needed.

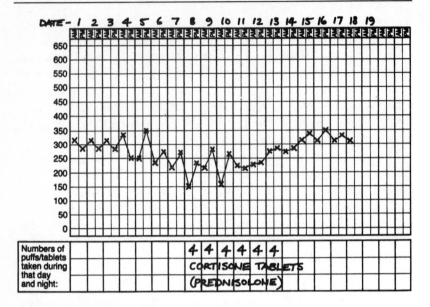

Figure 3.6   Peak flow chart showing an asthma attack. The readings decrease from day 5 to 8, and the gap between the morning and evening readings increases over this time.

Once you know your normal readings, the meter makes it easier to make changes in treatment and to decide whether you should contact your doctor or the hospital. There are some warning signs that an asthma attack may be coming, which we illustrate here with some examples.

- If the readings are dropping (see Figure 3.5). The dot shows the readings before relief inhalers (salbutamol) and the 'x' shows the reading after relief medication. In this chart the readings dropped slowly from the 12th to the morning of the 16th. Then suddenly they plummeted downwards on the evening of the 16th through the 17th. This man needed hospital admission on the 16th because his asthma was so bad.
- If the gap between morning and evening readings is widening (see Figure 3.6). This 7-year-old child's peak flow chart started off pretty level then from the 4th of the month the gap between the morning and evening readings starts to widen. The readings

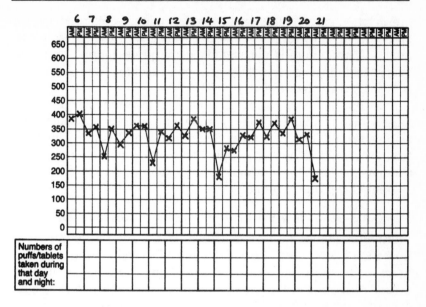

Figure 3.7   A chart showing early morning dipping of the peak flow. More (or different) treatment and medical help are needed urgently if this is happening.

change from 330 to 250 on the 4th, then from 250 to 300 on the 5th. The readings then drop from 270 on the evening of the 7th to 150 the following morning. The wide gap between the readings is a danger sign. This child needed prednisolone tablets (four a day) in addition to more of her usual inhalers to treat the attack.

- If there are some dips in the readings, in other words some readings are a lot lower than usual (see Figure 3.7). The early morning dips in peak flow on this chart on the 8th, 11th, 15th and 21st of the month were very serious warnings of uncontrolled asthma. This person needed more treatment, and the doctor was consulted urgently.

How do I obtain a peak flow meter?

Peak flow meters (Figure 3.1) are available on NHS prescription in the UK. Your general practitioner will be able to prescribe one for you. There are several different makes of meter, and your doctor's prescription should state exactly which meter is required, giving both the manufacturer's name and the type (low or standard range). If the make is not stated on the prescription, the pharmacist will dispense the cheapest one available. The cheapest is not necessarily the best!

Ask your doctor if you are in doubt about whether you should have a meter. Opinions differ over what proportion of people with asthma should have their own. Some health professionals believe that all should, others that only those with more troublesome asthma – perhaps those who require regular preventive treatment – should keep one at home.

I've got a peak flow meter, but what is a normal reading?

'Normal' readings are usually shown in a chart inside the peak flow meter box. They depend on your sex, height and age, but there is a big problem associated with them, which is that there is a very wide range of 'normal' readings for any particular height and age. For example, the normal 'chart' reading for a 3 foot 11 inch (120 cm) child lies between 120 and 300 litres per minute. This means that a reading anywhere between the two figures could be regarded as normal. So it would be quite possible to blow a reading that is 'normal' according to the chart, but is actually very low for that child. This is simply not very helpful. It is much more useful to establish your 'best ever' reading as your 'normal' reading. A daily peak flow diary card may help you to discover this best or 'normal' reading. This makes it easier to tell when your asthma is going out of control.

If the reading is dropping a long way below your best reading, then trouble is probably on the way.

The most important use of the peak flow meter is to see how much readings are changing (varying) from morning to evening, and from day to day. Everyone should know their own personal best reading, in order to be able to identify when asthma attacks are starting.

My child is 3 years old, and on regular asthma treatment. When can he start to use a peak flow meter effectively?

There is no particular age at which a child becomes able to use a meter (Figure 3.1). Some children are able to use them at four years of age and some are still struggling well past five or six years. If you can get consistent readings when your child is well, between attacks, then it is worth continuing with the readings. The great value of finding out his peak expiratory flow (PEF) levels when he is well is that it enables you to assess future attacks. By comparing the readings during symptoms with previous measurements when well, you will be able to decide more easily whether there is any need for increased medication or medical help.

There can be a disadvantage in trying to teach very young children how to blow peak flows. Sometimes they become confused between the action of breathing **in** to take their treatment, and blowing **out** to record their PEF. If this happens, and the result is that they do not take their treatment effectively, it is better to abandon the peak flow meter for a few months, until they can separate the two actions easily. The Windmill trainer is a new device available free from Clement Clarke International, and useful when teaching young children to blow into a peak flow meter properly.

Why do peak expiratory flow readings vary so much in the mornings and why do people with asthma have a 'morning dip'?

In this sense, 'morning dip' is nothing to do with a trip to the local swimming pool! Asthma is indeed worse during the early hours of the day, and PEF tends to be lowest at this time. This **drop** in peak flow is called a 'morning dip'. There are many theories about the cause of the morning dip, but no proof at the present time. Possible explanations include posture when asleep, leakage of acid from the gullet into the airways, low body steroid levels during the night, and even low levels of body growth hormone during the night. Many careful research studies have investigated this problem, but have not yet provided acceptable answers.

In practical terms, the size of the morning dip gives a good idea of how poorly controlled the asthma is. In people whose asthma is very well controlled there is little or no dip in the morning PEF reading. Treatment aims to remove the morning dip, and this is why it is best to make at least two measurements of PEF during each 24 hours. This helps us see how much morning dip there is. The readings are usually highest in the afternoon.

Some people have well controlled asthma but still experience large morning dips in their PEF. Extra treatments are required by these people; either one of the longer acting bronchodilator drugs – salmeterol xinafoate (Serevent) or eformoterol fumarate (Foradil and Oxis) – may also be an effective addition to preventer treatment.

I have two peak flow meters, one for home and one for my bag. If I use both at the same time I get different readings. For example, if one reads 530 litres per minute, the other reads 480 litres per minute. Does this matter?

No two meters are exactly the same. There are several types of peak flow meter (Figure 3.1), and a number of different manufacturers. Different meters often give readings that vary by 10% or more, even if they are of the same type and make. These differences are small, but may be important in individual cases. This can be very confusing for people with asthma, as well as for the doctors and nurses caring for them. It can be misleading to compare readings from home (on a prescribed meter) with the doctor's own meter in the surgery or outpatient clinic.

The ideal approach is to use exactly the same meter on each occasion. Since peak flow meters became available on prescription in the NHS, this has become possible for nearly everyone. It is best therefore to take your own peak flow meter when attending the clinic. If this is not practicable, then at least be aware that there can be an important difference between meters. In your own case, if you do find it necessary to have two meters, then the difference between the two should be consistent. As long as you are aware of the variation you can make allowances for it.

Self-management plans

What is a self-management plan?

Self-management plans have come very much to the fore in the past few years. The title is rather grand, but a self-management plan is simply an agreement between you and your doctor (or you and your doctor and asthma nurse) about the steps you can take to deal with your symptoms before calling for medical help. In this way you become much more involved in the day to day control of your condition, and can respond to changing needs for treatment.

These sorts of agreements have existed for years, of course, but the emphasis has changed recently in two important ways. Firstly, it is much more likely that plans will be written down. A range of cards, charts and booklets has been devised to enable the plan to be laid out clearly in writing. Secondly, in most cases except for young children, peak expiratory flow (PEF) readings will form an important part of the plan, so that at certain peak flow levels (which vary from person to person depending on a number of factors) changes in treatment are triggered. For example, your plan might say that you should start a course of prednisolone tablets if your PEF reading drops below 250, when normally it is between 480 and 520. In this case, you would start this course of treatment without needing to see your doctor first. (The figures and treatments we give here are only examples, and you should **not** use them. Discuss a similar plan with your own doctor.)

Some plans are quite complex, with a number of steps that may be taken, depending on changes in symptoms and PEF readings. Others are much more simple, for example saying 'if your PEF reading falls below 75% of your best reading, take two puffs of your reliever inhaler, and if you have not improved in 20 minutes, call your doctor'.

Research has shown that self-management plans work better if they are written down, and it is likely that they are more effective if PEF readings are used as well as just symptoms.

How do you work out the percentages on the self-management plans?

Calculating a percentage target for PEF is a useful way of guarding against uncontrolled asthma. The idea is to discover the best peak flow that you can achieve, and then to use this as a 'benchmark' or standard, against which action levels can be calculated.

If you take PEF readings regularly, when well and completely free of symptoms, you will soon establish what your usual best

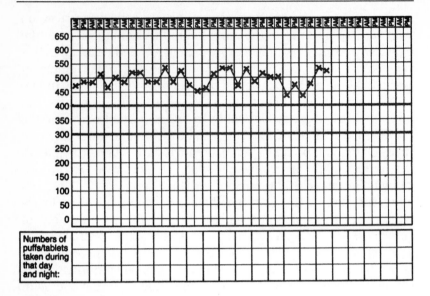

Figure 3.8   Peak flow chart showing 'normal' or 'best' readings around 500 litres per minute. Action lines have been drawn at 80% (500 × 0.8 = 400) and 60% (500 × 0.6 = 300).

reading is. Action levels for increasing treatment are calculated at certain percentages of this. A quick way to work out the percentages is to use a calculator and multiply your best readings by 0.1 for 10%, 0.2 for 20%, 0.3 for 30% and so on. This is all probably best explained by an example, using the chart in Figure 3.8. In this case, the person involved has a best PEF reading of 500. Two action levels are calculated.

1 An 80% level (multiply the best reading of 500 by 0.8):
$$500 \times 0.8 = 400$$
2 A 60% level (multiply the best reading of 500 by 0.6):
$$500 \times 0.6 = 300$$

Two lines are drawn on the chart at these 80% and 60% levels, and used as guidelines. If the PEF readings stay above the top line (80% of best) then the asthma is well controlled, and treatment is not changed. If the readings drop towards the top line, usual treatment needs to be increased (see Figure 3.9). If the readings

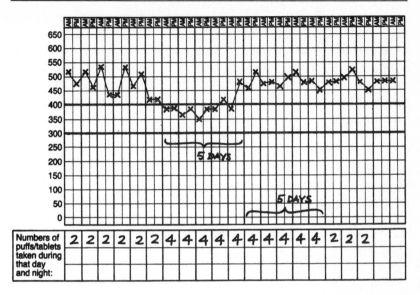

Figure 3.9   Chart showing action lines. If the readings drop below the
first line, the inhaled steroids (preventers) should be doubled until the
readings have remained normal for the same number of days it took to
get better.

drop towards the bottom line (60% of best) then urgent action is
needed. Extra doses of relief medication should be taken straight
away, and prednisolone tablets are probably needed. Urgent
medical advice may also be needed at this point.

These two levels of action (80% and 60% of best readings) are
probably the two used most commonly, but the great advantage of
such plans is that they can be made to suit the individual. Some
people need more than two action levels because they take a large
number of treatments. Some people do better with different action
levels. It is a case of you and the health professionals working
together to decide on the most suitable plan for you. The guiding
principle, however, is that it is essential to know the best reading
that you can achieve.

How long should you continue to take your preventers at the
higher dose? The peak flow chart may be helpful in answering this
question. Some people's asthma follows a set pattern where the

person knows how long their asthma episodes usually last. These people will usually know when it is safe to reduce the dose and go back to the previous levels. Another way of reducing the dose is to count how many days it took from the time your PEF readings dropped below the line, up until the day when they reached your previous best levels. Then simply carry on taking the higher dose for the same number of days. For example, look at the chart in Figure 3.9 where the normal (best ever) peak flow is about 500. So two action lines have been drawn at 400 (80%) and 300 (60%). This person doubled his inhaled steroid puffs from two to four in the morning and evening. He continued at this dose until the readings returned to the normal level. He then counted how many days it took him to get better (five days). Then he continued at the double dose for the same number of days, i.e. for another five days after he got better.

An agreed holiday self-management plan to deal with an emergency is extremely helpful, and here is an example.

If your PEF drops below 60% of your normal or best previous levels there are three things to do.

- Don't panic.
- Take a lot of the reliever drugs (either Bricanyl – generic name terbutaline sulphate; or Ventolin Evohaler – generic name salbutamol). In an emergency take one puff every 10 seconds until you feel better (you may need 15–30 puffs).
- Take a dose of prednisolone tablets. Agree an emergency dose of these cortisone tablets with your doctor before going away on holiday.

This is merely an example; you should decide individual drugs and doses with your own doctor.

Altering treatment

Am I allowed to alter my treatment, or should my doctor always do this?

Nearly all doctors and nurses who have an interest in asthma do aim to help their patients become expert in managing their own asthma. Thus, a major role for the health professional is to enable people with asthma to take care of their asthma themselves, while consulting with them regularly to reinforce this independence. This means that a clear self-management plan must be agreed, and this will usually include the following:

• Extra medication will be needed if exposure to known triggers is expected.
• Recognition of the common symptoms of developing asthma will lead to an increase in medication. If this helps, the dose will be continued according to the self-management plan.
• It is common to continue at the increased dose for a while after recovery takes place. The length of time will vary from person to person and between different episodes of asthma.
• There are no fixed rules, only guidelines. Use of peak flow charts in these circumstances is very helpful.
• If the increased medication fails to help, a policy for obtaining urgent medical help is set out.

In our jargon, this type of approach is called 'guided self-management', and means that you can alter your treatment with changing symptoms, or changing peak expiratory flow, according to your agreed plan. Your doctor must also, of course, be available when problems arise and your self-treatment is not working. It should not be a case of losing your access to medical advice because you want to take charge of your own condition.

There is a section on *Self-management plans* earlier in this chapter.

How long do I need to take my medicine for?

This depends largely on your age. Asthma is generally a lifelong condition, and people do not outgrow their asthmatic tendency. However, the disease often goes quiet for a while, perhaps for many years, only to flare up again after exposure to a trigger, or more often for no apparent reason. Because of this you need to take continuous treatment aimed at preventing the inflammation of asthma. Your treatment could be increased or decreased depending on your symptoms and your PEF readings. If your asthma has gone quiet (into remission), your treatment might be reduced or even stopped (using peak flow charts for guidance) and only resumed if your symptoms come back.

Having started asthma treatment most doctors would advise that children continue taking medication for at least a year. The main factor is the severity of the asthma. If after a year of treatment, the asthma is very mild and there are few symptoms or attacks, then therapy might be stopped. In older children, this is best done with the help of a peak flow chart which provides warning of uncontrolled asthma.

In adults asthma treatment is usually for life. However, some adults only get short episodes of asthma and once these have cleared up, with little variation of the PEF, it is worth stopping the treatment. The use of a peak flow chart in this situation is very helpful in deciding whether treatment should be resumed.

Do I have to stay on Becotide forever?

Like the answer to the previous question, this depends mainly on your age! Adults usually need to remain on preventive treatment for life. In children, most doctors would advise treatment for at least a year or so. Then, using a regular daily peak flow chart to make sure that all is well, treatment might be stopped, and restarted only if the readings vary by more than 15%. Such children may not have any further trouble from their asthma, but the family should be aware that it could flare up after a time (which may be a number of years). In pre-school children, PEF readings can be difficult to obtain, and unreliable.

If prescribed drugs are taken regularly, is it ever possible to cut down the dosage, and in time give up taking drugs altogether?

Yes, it is possible. As a rough and ready rule, the longer your asthma symptoms have been kept under good control by treatment, the less likely it is that symptoms will come back if you reduce your treatment. This means we have to steer a course between carrying on with a treatment that is very effective, and reducing the dose. Nobody knows the answer with any certainty. Some people feel that symptoms should be controlled for a year before treatment is reduced ('stepped down' in current jargon). Others believe that dosages can be reduced much sooner. Doctors vary, and so do patients!

Regular checking with a peak flow meter makes it easier to adjust your treatment. If you have few symptoms and your peak flow readings vary only slightly from morning to evening, then it is probably safe to reduce your medication. It would be advisable to discuss this question with your doctor or asthma nurse.

Can we decrease our son's medication? He has just had his seventh birthday, and has been well for two months.

Possibly – discuss it with your doctor or asthma nurse. Two months without problems is very encouraging, but it may be a little soon to adjust his treatment. Somewhere between three to six months is preferable. This is where peak flow meters are very helpful. A chart should show whether it is safe to decrease his medication. A level peak flow chart such as the one in Figure 3.4 would indicate that his asthma is well controlled. The graph is almost a straight line. In this case you could try reducing his medication, and then see what happens to the PEF. If the readings stay level without going up and down too much and there are no symptoms, then it is safe to continue on the lower dose. If the readings do begin to vary, then the control of asthma is being lost, and the previous dose should be taken again.

As a rule of thumb his readings should not go up or down by more than 15%. The formula to calculate this change (variation) is:

$$\frac{\text{Highest} - \text{Lowest reading}}{\text{Highest}} \times 100 = \% \text{ change of peak flow}$$

If the change is greater than 15% then the variation is too high and his asthma is out of control. For example, if his highest reading during the week is 400 and the lowest is 300, the peak flow variation is therefore 25%. This is a lot higher than 15%, and would indicate that his asthma is quite badly out of control.

As long as his peak flow readings don't go up or down by more than 15% then it is safe for him to stay on the lower dose. In a few more months it may be possible to make another reduction in the treatment.

Is it better for me to put up with my asthma, and not take any drugs?

No, and if putting up with asthma means that you are having symptoms then the answer is definitely no. The presence of symptoms of asthma probably means the presence of inflammation of the airways. Asthma inflammation is an ongoing process which may damage the lungs. The presence of inflammation may also make the asthma more liable to flare up and cause an attack. We feel that people whose asthma is causing them symptoms should be taking regular anti-asthma medication aimed at healing the underlying inflammation. Such preventer drugs include beclomethasone dipropionate (Becotide), budesonide (Pulmicort), fluticasone propionate (Flixotide), nedocromil sodium (Tilade) and sodium cromoglycate (Intal).

When can I stop my steroids after an attack?

The best way to decide this is with the help of a peak flow meter and a daily chart. Most doctors today accept that people with asthma can follow a self-management plan, once this has been agreed. There is a section on *Self-management plans* earlier in this chapter, but the basic guidelines for such a plan are as follows.

- The usual PEF reading is taken as the normal reading. People who have their own meters will usually have a good idea of their normal readings.
- When the peak expiratory flow drops below 50–60% of the normal reading, the person starts a course of steroid tablets. The dose is usually 20–30 milligrams per day for children, depending on what your doctor advises in discussion, and 30–60 milligrams per day in adults.
- The tablets are continued at this daily dose until the peak flow reaches the normal value for that person. Then the daily dose is halved and continued for the same number of days it took for the peak flow to reach normal levels. It is important to keep on with the tablets until after a good response has been achieved.

An example may help to explain all this more clearly. Figure 3.10

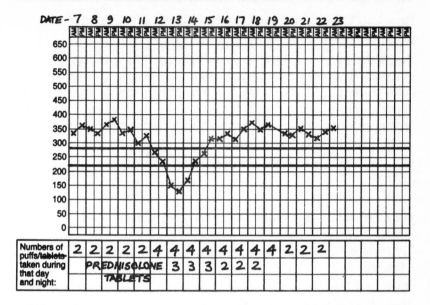

Figure 3.10 Peak flow chart showing an asthma attack that has improved. The readings came back to normal after self-treatment with increased inhalers and steroid tablets when they dropped below the two action lines.

shows the chart of a child whose parents managed to treat an asthma attack successfully. The inhaled steroid dose was doubled from two to four puffs morning and evening when the peak flow dropped below the 80% action line on the 12th. On the 13th, when the peak flow dropped below the 60% line, they then started 15 milligrams (three 5 milligram tablets) daily of prednisolone tablets (as previously agreed with their doctor). This dose was continued until the readings came back to normal, above the top line. The parents counted the number of days it took their child to get better (three days). They then continued at a reduced dose of two tablets daily for the same number (three) of days. **This plan had been previously agreed between the family and the doctor**. It is safe to follow this as long as the asthma is improving. It is clear from the chart that the child was improving. If this had not been the case medical help would have been required urgently.

How can I recognize that my treatment is working?

When your symptoms have improved and your peak flow chart has returned towards normal, your treatment is working. The use of a daily peak flow chart is most helpful when new treatment has been started or when the dose of existing treatment is increased. Signs of improvement on the chart are, firstly, that your readings are fairly constant and they don't vary much from morning to evening, and from day to day, and secondly that your readings are increasing towards your 'normal' or best values.

Recognizing uncontrolled asthma

My 'puffer' inhaler doesn't work any more. What is wrong with it?

We assume that you are using your inhaler correctly in the first place. If so there could still be several reasons for this. It could be that the hole through which the drug is delivered has become blocked with deposits of drug particles. If you breathe in and out of the inhaler mouth several times before depressing the canister, it is more likely to become blocked because of condensation. It is important to clean the inhaler regularly as is recommended and described in the patient information leaflet dispensed with the inhaler.

Another more obvious reason for it not to 'work' any more is that it could be empty! It is not always easy to tell how much remains in the canister. Many people learn how to measure this by shaking the canister gently, and getting a feel for how much is left. It is much easier to tell when one of the new CFC-free puffers is empty – they simply stop working. Once the new CFC-free metered dose inhalers (puffers) are used more widely, the problem will be largely resolved.

Sometimes people say (and feel) that their inhaler is not working when in fact there is nothing wrong with it. There are two important explanations for this. The person may be confused about the type of inhaler they are using – for example between a preventer and a reliever. Because it is effective as a preventer rather than giving instant relief, the steroid inhaler may appear not to 'work'. Some people misunderstand the way in which pre-venters are supposed to help their asthma, and decide that they are of no help. Most importantly, however, people sometimes feel, correctly, that their reliever inhaler is not working as it usually does because their asthma is getting worse. This is the most important sign of uncontrolled asthma.

How will I recognize that the treatment is not working, and more or different treatment is needed?

Needing more relief medication and a worsening peak flow chart are the two most important clues that you need extra treatment. Anyone who requires Ventolin or Airomir (salbutamol) or Bricanyl (terbutaline) more than once a day should really be taking a reg-ular preventer drug. So an increased need for Ventolin or Bricanyl serves as a warning that your asthma is out of control and that extra medication is necessary. This information can be used as follows.

- If your asthma is usually mild, only requiring a reliever drug when you get symptoms, and you find that you need to use this reliever drug more than once a day, then a regular preventer drug is required.
- If you are already using one of the preventer drugs, and you find that you need to use your reliever drug more than once a day, then your dose of preventer drug needs to be increased.
- If you need to use the reliever drug more than every four hours **whatever your treatment** – in other words the effect of your reliever drug is lasting less than four hours – then THIS IS IMPORTANT – MEDICAL ADVICE IS NEEDED URGENTLY.

The need for using extra doses of the reliever drugs can therefore be used practically. You can use this information to provide your doctor or asthma nurse with information to add new preventive medication, to adjust your own medication, and to help you recognize when to call for help.

Why can asthma attacks be so unpredictable?

Sometimes asthma attacks **are** unpredictable, and in these cases urgent self-treatment should be started. In some people these unpredictable attacks can be very severe and then it is a good idea to carry spare supplies of emergency asthma drugs to counter them. Precisely because they are unpredictable, it is difficult for us to explain exactly why they occur! All we can say is that asthma is a very variable condition, and that sometimes it takes a combination of triggers, or circumstances, to spark off an attack. Perhaps someone is allergic to cats, but nine times out of ten they do not get asthma on meeting a cat. Suppose that on the tenth occasion they are very stressed, or they have just started a cold, or have just moved house and inhaled lots of dust. These extra circumstances may be enough to set off an attack when they come into contact with the cat.

More often, asthma is very predictable, but people are not aware of it. For example some people continue to go into stables even though the hay and the horses are the triggers for their attacks. Others insist on smoking even though this makes their asthma worse. By avoiding known personal trigger factors many 'unpredictable' asthma attacks may be prevented.

How can I prevent an asthma attack?

Some asthma attacks cannot be prevented, yet most can. The key to preventing attacks is to avoid your known trigger factors if at all possible and to recognize your early warning signs. Take extra treatment as soon as possible, and call for medical help if this does not work. Most severe attacks can be prevented by these actions. You should discuss your own circumstances and actions with your doctor or asthma nurse, but these are the things to look out for: increased symptoms; lowered peak expiratory flow readings (PEFs); an increase in the gap between the morning and evening readings; or steadily dropping levels of PEF. These are all important signs of uncontrolled asthma. The charts in the section on **Peak flow monitoring** earlier in this chapter show examples of these changes.

What should I do if my son panics and becomes breathless?

Stay calm, and try to encourage him to stay calm. This is not easy, but the more you panic, the worse he is likely to become. Next, give him a high dose of reliever drug (15–30 puffs of Ventolin Evohaler, Bricanyl or Airomir). This action is perfectly safe, and may be necessary to open up the airways. If you have a spacer device (Aerochamber, Volumatic or Nebuhaler – Figures 2.9–2.10) available it is best to give the drug using this, giving one puff every 10 seconds. If not, any sort of emergency chamber, such as a paper or plastic cup, or even a paper bag, will do (see Figure 2.14). Failing that, simply fire the inhaler into his mouth as he breathes. It is better to get a small amount of the drug into his airways than none at all. It is important that only one puff is squirted into the spacer at a time. In other words, puff once just before the person breathes in, wait until they have breathed in two or three times and then puff again.

If this does not help within minutes, then you have an emergency requiring urgent medical help. If this cannot be obtained, he should be taken immediately to the nearest casualty (Accident and Emergency) department – by ambulance if possible. Ambulances carry oxygen, and can get to hospital quickly.

If you have them available, give him prednisolone tablets before you go to hospital (that is, the dose that has previously been agreed with your doctor).

Should I carry an inhaler with me during the day, even if I expect to use it only at both ends of the day?

This is going to depend on which type of inhaler you are talking about. The preventer inhalers that are usually prescribed twice daily are the inhaled steroids (e.g. Becotide, Pulmicort, Flixotide) and these do not need to be carried around with you during the day. The reason for this is that they will not give you immediate relief from symptoms and so are not used 'on demand'.

Reliever inhalers (e.g. Ventolin, Bricanyl, Airomir) are for immediate relief of symptoms, and should be kept with you at all times.

The two other types of inhalers which may have been prescribed twice a day are Serevent (salmeterol xinafoate) and Oxivent. Neither of these needs to be carried with you as, again, they are not intended to be used more than twice daily.

4
Life with Asthma

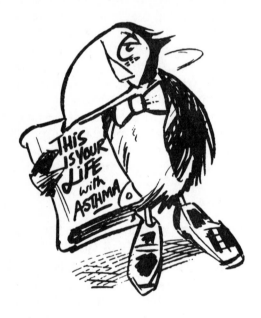

Introduction

This chapter deals with some of those very practical questions which have been posed by people with asthma concerning their daily lives. As with other chapters there are several sections, but all deal with particular aspects of the environment in which we live, from home problems to holidays in the Alps. There is much controversy about the apparent increase over the past 20 years in the numbers of people who have asthma. It does appear that there has been a significant increase in the proportion of children with asthma, and there is a school of thought that this is due to changes in our environment, particularly the effects of pollution.

Many women with asthma have problems related either to pregnancy or to their periods. For the latter, most questions referred to worsening asthma during periods or just before. This is a well recognized problem. Clearly the body sex hormones have some influence over asthma. Changes occur not only in pregnancy and periods but also during puberty. This is an interesting area which demands more research.

Asthma in the workplace was given great prominence during 1991 when a woman won industrial compensation from her employers because of the adverse effects on her asthma of cigarette smoke in her work environment. Holidays should be a time for you to enjoy yourself, rather than thinking about your asthma, but a little forward planning with respect to your asthma can save an awful lot of misery resulting from acute attacks in far away places.

Following the enormous changes to the National Health Service during 1990 and 1991 there has been much concern about the costs of treatment for asthma. At the time of going to press we know of no circumstances where the correct treatment for asthma has been justifiably withheld on the grounds of cost. There is considerable pressure on doctors to reduce prescribing costs wherever possible. Good asthma treatments are not cheap, but if they improve short- and long-term health of people with asthma, and avoid expensive hospital admissions, there can be no justification for withholding them.

Everyday life

Can someone's asthma be affected by their social background?

Some studies have shown that asthma is more common in families with one or two children compared with larger families. A linked finding suggests that children from higher socioeconomic groups are more prone to asthma. Why this happens is not entirely clear

at present but research has come up with one interesting suggestion. This shows that the youngest children in large families
seem more likely to catch lots of colds and respiratory infections
in early childhood from their older brothers and sisters. This
seems to boost their immune systems, so that they are less likely
to develop allergic problems like hay fever. Children in small
families seem less likely to catch these early infections, but more
likely to suffer from allergic conditions, which we know are
strongly associated with asthma.

Another important factor in the social background is whether
the family contains smokers. We know that children who are
exposed to smoke are more likely to suffer from asthma. This
applies to smoking by parents and other members of the family.
Smoking in pregnancy also appears to have an unfavourable effect
on the unborn baby. We do not understand why this happens but
the important message to parents is 'Don't smoke', it is harmful for
your children.

Why is my asthma at its worst when I carry heavy shopping?

Any strenuous exercise may trigger asthma symptoms, and
carrying shopping is just one example of this. If exercise only
makes your asthma worse on occasions such as this, you could
prevent it by taking an extra dose of reliever medication just
before the activity in question. If, however, this is a more regular
problem and your asthma gets bad every time you exercise, then
you probably need more preventer medication. The clue to
needing more preventer drug is when a dose of reliever medication is needed to help symptoms at least once every day. Discuss
this with your doctor or asthma nurse.

A peak flow diary card can help in finding the right dose to
prevent symptoms (we make no apology for repeating this
advice!). If your morning and evening readings differ by a lot
(more than 15%) then you should increase your medication dose
every few days until your readings no longer vary by so much from
morning to evening. Once you reach the correct dose, your chart
will appear almost flat. Figure 1.5 shows an example of a chart
where the readings gradually improve after treatment; Figure 3.4
shows the chart of someone with well controlled asthma.

Why is asthma often bad at night?

This is another simple question with a complex answer! In short, nobody knows for sure. There are various theories, and these have been the subject of much interest and research.

Waking at night with asthma is very common, very unpleasant and can be terrifying. Only fairly recently have doctors realized how frequent and important night-time asthma really is. Some of the possible reasons include: how you lie when you are asleep; dust and house dust mites in the bedding; low levels of certain body hormones at night (particularly cortisol); increased acid production by the stomach; changes in air and body temperature; and loss of effect of asthma drugs taken earlier in the day. Quite a list, although most have been ruled out as major causes.

Perhaps most crucial amongst them is the change that takes place in the body's natural rhythms during the night. All of us (whether or not we have asthma) have a lung function rhythm within a 24-hour period. This is highest at around 4.00pm and lowest at around 4.00am. In poorly controlled asthma the low point is much more marked, and breathing can worsen dramatically in the early morning. This low point matches the low point for hormones produced by the body, and the two are probably connected. There is still much to learn about asthma at night. One thing we can say is that good day-time control leads to improvements in night-time asthma.

I sometimes wheeze when I go near a dog, house dust etc. Is this an allergy, or asthma?

It is probably both. The allergic reaction to the trigger (dog, dust etc.) starts off the asthma attack. As well as the asthma there may well be other signs of allergy, particularly streaming nose and sneezing, and itchy eyes.

Why do I wheeze when I go into a warm house from the cold outside?

Usually it happens the other way round. Cold air is a well known trigger of asthma symptoms, and a transfer from a warm house to the open air in the winter frequently makes people cough and wheeze. It may be that your symptoms begin outside in the cold, but become more noticeable when you get indoors. However, a change in temperature from cold to warm can also spark off an attack in some people. You may be one of these people or there may also be other allergens in the warm house that trigger your symptoms. These are most likely to be dusts, moulds or animal hairs.

Why do I feel uncomfortable in gas central heating and feel better when cool?

You are not alone in experiencing this problem, and other people have noticed that their asthma gets unaccountably worse in centrally heated houses. We do know that warm, centrally heated homes are ideal for the house dust mite population. They love to bask in the warmth, and they multiply in great quantities. If there are any gas fumes from the boiler this could also increase your discomfort. Even during winter months when the central heating is needed most it is a good idea to have some outside air circulating in the house.

Another possibility is that a change of air temperature from the cool outside to the warm inside can trigger symptoms when your asthma is not very well controlled. One final question – is there cigarette smoke in the atmosphere? If so, this is more likely to cause problems than the central heating.

At the beginning of the winter months, when the central heating is switched on, why do my nasal passages feel very tickly, and what shall I do about it?

This condition is called rhinitis, and many people with asthma also are sufferers from it. There are two likely explanations for these symptoms. One is allergy to the house dust mite, and the other is the onset of cold winter weather.

In allergic rhinitis the lining of the nasal passages reacts to trigger factors (allergens). The reaction may be a tickly sensation, a feeling of being blocked or even a runny nose with frequent sneezing. There are many possible allergens, but the best known example is grass pollen – the cause of hay fever. In your case, house dust mite allergy is the most likely cause. Although the house dust mite can cause problems throughout the year, the numbers are at their highest in the early winter months. Switching on the central heating can also give a boost to their numbers by raising the temperature.

Cold weather is another trigger factor for rhinitis. This is not true allergy, but is generally called vasomotor rhinitis. Cold air causes a reaction in the lining of the nose, with results similar to allergy.

If your rhinitis is very troublesome, we suggest that you talk to your doctor about it. There are several highly effective treatments available, but most of them are on prescription.

Is it all right to buy a cough medicine for my tickly cough when I have inhalers for my asthma?

We would not recommend it, and would go so far as to say it would be a waste of money. There is really no place for cough medicines in the treatment of asthma since there is no evidence that they are able to stop the coughing caused by asthma. The use of cough medicines only serves to delay proper anti-asthma treatment. Your tickly cough is almost certainly a sign that the asthma is not sufficiently controlled by the treatment you are taking. This is extremely important. Rather than move on to a useless treatment such as a cough medicine, you should increase your inhalers, or talk to your doctor or asthma nurse about adjusting your treatment.

Asthma symptoms such as tickly coughs may develop into full blown asthma attacks if they are not treated properly, and turning to a cough mixture will not help.

Can I give blood?

In general, anyone who requires regular prescribed medication cannot be accepted as a blood donor (this applies to everyone who takes regular medicines, not just those with asthma). The only way round this situation would be for you to stop your preventive treatment for a few days before giving blood. We do not recommend this, as it is potentially harmful. If, however, you only need to take occasional reliever treatment such as Ventolin or Bricanyl, you will be accepted as a donor. These are the guidelines of the National Blood Transfusion Service about people with asthma giving blood. They may, however, be interpreted differently by individual transfusion centres, and so it might be advisable to contact your local transfusion centre directly to confirm our advice regarding your suitability as a donor.

Are people with asthma more at risk than other people when given a general anaesthetic?

The answer to this is no – providing that your asthma is well controlled. Your lungs need to be in as good a condition as possible and the airways unrestricted. If you know you are going to be given an anaesthetic, then it would be well worth you doing a series of peak flow measurements, if possible, for about two weeks beforehand (see the section on *Peak flow expiratory monitoring* in Chapter 3 for more details about these). You can then check that your asthma is well controlled. If this is not the case, an early consultation with your doctor should be arranged, rather than one just before your operation.

It is obviously important that the anaesthetist knows that the patient has asthma, so that they can take any extra steps that might be necessary. In some hospitals the anaesthetist will ask those with asthma to use a nebulizer before they are given the anaesthetic. This ensures that the airways are as fully dilated as possible. Remember, the anaesthetist is in a very good position to check and put right any breathing problems during anaesthesia.

People with chronic severe asthma, and those with other lung conditions as well as asthma, are at much greater risk when given an anaesthetic than someone whose asthma is well controlled. Nowadays the range of operations which can be performed under a local anaesthetic is much greater, and so general anaesthetics need to be given less often to people at high risk.

I have asthma. Is it safe for me to have an operation?

There is no reason why you, or anyone else who has asthma, should not have an operation. Many surgical operations require a general anaesthetic, and we have discussed this in detail in the previous question.

It is very important to continue your asthma treatment postoperatively. Some hospitals take away the patient's own inhaler device and substitute it with a different type. If this is the case, do check that you know how to use the new inhaler. Some hospitals only dispense the metered dose inhaler – not everyone is able to use this device, and careful instruction is needed. If you are not happy with your new treatment do see your GP when you leave hospital.

Will asthma affect my son's future regarding getting insurance?

This depends on the severity of his asthma and the type of insurance he requires. Life insurance may be more difficult to obtain at usual premiums than endowment insurance. People with the most severe asthma and those requiring long-term treatment are likely to receive insurance quotations with extra loading on their premiums. However, some companies are more sympathetic than others, and there is a wide variety of companies to choose from. It is therefore advisable to shop around for the best buy. An independent insurance broker is best placed to do this on your son's behalf because they are not tied to any one company. If you do receive a 'loaded' quotation from a company, a letter from your son's GP to the company, asking for an explanation, may be of help in lowering the premium.

In every application for insurance, the GP is asked to provide a medical report for the insurance company. As long as the person involved has signed a consent form, the GP will disclose relevant medical information to the insurance company. This information may help or hinder the person's chances of obtaining a low premium. For example, someone who fails to take regular treatment for asthma despite medical advice may be loaded as a result of the disclosure of this information. On the other hand, someone who is careful, and attends regularly for check-ups may get a lower premium from the company.

Your son is entitled to see the report before it is sent to the company. He may ask for it to be altered if he disagrees with it, but the doctor is obliged to tell the insurance company that alterations have been made.

Smoking

I have heard that smoking doesn't affect asthma – is that true?

No! This may be some sort of folklore which goes back to the days when asthma cigarettes (which contained herbs, not nicotine and tar) were sold as treatments for the condition. This was a very early form of inhaled treatment!

In fact there is very strong evidence now that asthma is made worse in the presence of cigarette smoke. This applies particularly to children, who may have to suffer in smoky atmospheres through no fault of their own.

A famous recent case, in which a female asthma sufferer won industrial compensation because of the harmful effects of involuntary smoking on her condition, has heightened public appreciation of this problem. Increasingly, workplaces are becoming non-smoking areas because the hazards of involuntary smoking are becoming clear.

Perhaps even more importantly, we are now seeing evidence that an increase in smoking amongst pregnant women and mothers is causing the development of asthma symptoms in their children later on in childhood.

How can I stop my husband smoking in front of the children?

Evidence for the harmful effects of cigarette smoke on children's asthma is increasing.

- Infants exposed passively to cigarette smoke suffer from more wheezing illness during the first year of life than infants who are not exposed.
- Lung growth and lung function in children whose parents smoke are not as good as in those whose parents do not smoke.
- Cigarette smoke is a trigger factor for asthma attacks.

The problem is particularly bad for children with asthma whose parent(s) or relatives smoke at home. Research suggests children whose mothers smoke suffer most, and that this is far worse for those children who are at home all day rather than away at school or nursery. So the problem is clearly related to the length of time the child spends with a smoker.

Parents who smoke are therefore putting their children's health at risk, both in the short term and in the long term. We know of no guaranteed way to solve your particular problem. Often people are simply unaware of the risks posed by involuntary smoking. Perhaps if you can convince your husband of these facts he might be prepared to smoke away from areas of direct contact with your children.

How can I ask people in my work environment to stop smoking?

It has been recognized for some time that exposure to tobacco smoke can cause discomfort and irritation, particularly to those who already have a chest problem such as asthma. There is no doubt that when smokers and non-smokers share the same room, non-smokers cannot avoid inhaling some environmental tobacco smoke as they breathe – this is called involuntary or passive smoking. The tobacco smoke concerned is mainly the 'sidestream' smoke from burning cigarettes, cigars or pipe tobacco but there is also some smoke exhaled by smokers. Tobacco smoke contains various substances that can trigger unpleasant asthma symptoms.

It is not easy to impose a complete ban on smoking at work. Proper consultation should take place with all the people involved, as simply imposing measures to control involuntary smoking can lead to resentment among smokers, and problems in enforcing the non-smoking rule. However, limiting or preventing smoking by an agreed and carefully implemented policy may improve employee morale, reduce arguments between smokers and non-smokers, reduce time lost through sickness, and even decrease cleaning bills! Perhaps you could suggest that smoking is limited to certain areas of your workplace. This is a perfectly reasonable request, and you should not feel you are being difficult or demanding. Perhaps you could join other non-smokers at your place of work and act together in making your request. After all, it is not only people with asthma who are keen to see this sort of control on places for smoking.

Sex, pregnancy and periods

Asthma seems to interfere with my sex life – why?

Although asthma is such a common condition it is not a frequent cause of sexual difficulties. However, if asthma does occur during sex it can cause problems. Symptoms can be brought on in several different ways. Firstly, by exertion. In these cases the use of a reliever drug such as Ventolin, Bricanyl or Airomir before inter-course can prevent such an attack. Secondly, movement in bed can sometimes cause large amounts of allergens to be released from the bed clothes, and this can trigger wheezing. Thirdly (and only rarely) a woman can be allergic to her partner's semen (sperm), and can develop a generalized allergic reaction which may include asthma. This can happen within a few minutes of intercourse, or several hours or days later. Whereas it is easy to associate the immediate reaction with sexual intercourse, it is much more difficult to identify the late reaction. The use of a condom can be an effective temporary measure, and can also be used to check that the diagnosis is correct. However, some types of condoms can themselves cause local allergic reactions, and so a low allergenic condom such as a Durex Allergy should be used. Women with this rare problem may be successfully desensitized by specialist treatment.

As far as we are aware drugs used in the treatment of asthma do not impair sexual desire or responses.

Does the oral contraceptive pill weaken the effects of doses of Ventolin or Becotide?

No!

What effect does being pregnant tend to have on asthma?

Pregnancy has a variable effect on asthma. Research has shown that for some women their asthma actually improves during pregnancy. These may be those women whose asthma tends to get worse during the week before their periods. The message from research is that around 40% of women require more treatment to control their asthma during pregnancy, around 40% keep to the same treatment and around 20% actually need less. All recent studies show that the health of a newborn baby is unaffected by whether or not the mother has asthma.

Any risk that there is for the baby during pregnancy comes from severe acute attacks. These may cause a shortage of oxygen which may be dangerous, for both the mother and her growing baby. This may result in smaller babies and even stillbirth in severe asthma attacks, though the latter is extremely rare. The preventer drugs (Becotide, Pulmicort, Flixotide, Intal and Tilade) are safe in pregnancy and are important in preventing such asthma attacks (see next question).

I've just been told I am pregnant – can I take my medication?

Yes, your medication can and indeed should be taken, provided you are taking it through the inhaled route. In the first three months of pregnancy, the general rule is to take no drugs by mouth (i.e. tablets or syrup) unless they are really necessary. Your

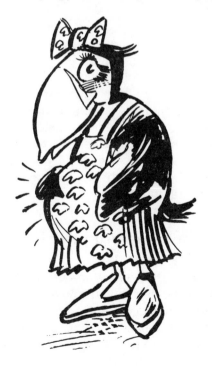

doctor can advise you about this. Drugs for asthma, taken by inhaler, are generally safe during all stages of pregnancy, whereas uncontrolled asthma is not. It is most important for you to try and control asthma well during your pregnancy. The main risk to your baby if you have severe attacks is that he or she may be born underweight, but there is a tiny, but real, risk of death of the baby in a very severe attack.

Because of this there is a good case to be made for regular peak flow monitoring in pregnancy in order to tell at an early stage when asthma is getting worse.

Will I get breathing difficulties in labour?

For all women at the end of pregnancy, the size of the uterus (womb), which contains the baby and all the fluid surrounding it, takes up a lot of extra space in the abdomen. This causes pressure, which pushes upwards on to the diaphragm, and squeezes the lungs. This results in breathing being slightly more difficult for all woman in late pregnancy and in labour. As long as your asthma is well controlled, your breathing should be no different from any other woman in labour. If your asthma is bad, then an extra strain will be placed on your breathing, and you may well notice problems. Talk to your doctor if you are worried about your asthma control in the later stages of your pregnancy.

The anxiety and excitement which occur when labour begins may result in you forgetting to take your asthma inhalers, or they may be left at home in the rush to get to hospital. It is a good idea to pack an extra inhaler in your maternity suitcase to avoid this. You can also help prevent breathing problems in labour by using the breathing exercises you have been taught at antenatal classes, and by taking your asthma medication regularly.

Is it OK for me to breastfeed while taking Ventolin and Becotide inhalers?

Yes! In standard doses these drugs are absorbed into your system in such microscopic amounts that the quantity appearing in breast milk will be almost undetectable. Using a spacer device to take your medication (a Volumatic – Figure 2.10 – for Becotide and Flixotide; and a Nebuhaler – Figure 2.11 – for Pulmicort) will reduce even further the amounts of the drugs swallowed and absorbed. This all but removes the chance of drugs appearing in your breast milk.

Will breastfeeding reduce the likelihood of my baby developing asthma, or its severity?

It would seem likely, on grounds of common sense and logic, that breastfeeding during the first few months of life (because it is a good thing generally) should reduce the chances of a child developing asthma (and other allergic diseases). The exposure to allergens found in cow's milk is also avoided. Some, but not all, research studies have not confirmed this for asthma. On the other hand, the evidence is quite strong that breastfeeding protects against development of atopic eczema when there is a family history of the condition. Breastfeeding needs to continue for around six months to reduce the chances of the baby becoming allergic to cow's milk, and then developing eczema.

By and large we believe that, with respect to asthma and allergies, it is much better for babies to be breastfed if possible, particularly where one or both parents are atopic or have asthma.

Could my periods have anything to do with my asthma?

Quite possibly, as it is likely that the menstrual cycle has an effect on asthma in many women. Research has shown that in some women asthma gets worse during the week before a period. This link between the premenstrual phase and asthma symptoms seems to be more pronounced in women with severe asthma. The problem here is that the more severe the asthma, the more frequent the attacks are likely to be. Asthma attacks may happen at any time of the month, but it may appear that they are worse just before the periods.

There is no convincing scientific evidence that periods themselves cause attacks of asthma. Some people are allergic to aspirin. Therefore aspirin and similar drugs (NSAIDs such as Nurofen, ibuprofen; Ponstan, mefenamic acid) used for period pain may induce an asthma attack. These drugs are best avoided (especially if you have nasal polyps) and, if they are used, peak expiratory flow monitoring may be helpful to detect danger signs (see *Self-management plans section* in Chapter 3). If you do take regular medication for period pain check, with your doctor.

The best way to test for a link between asthma and periods in your own case is to keep a regular record of your peak expiratory flow readings. If there is a consistent fall in readings around or before your period, then that is strong evidence to support your suspicions. If so, it would be sensible to increase your preventer treatment during the week before falls in peak flow are expected.

Once a month I've ended up in hospital, back on steroids, and being nebulized. This is because of my periods. Why?

There is some evidence suggesting that there is a link between asthma and periods. A high proportion of women with asthma report that their asthma becomes worse in the later part of their cycle or at the start of menstruation, although not often as severely as in your case. How the female hormone factors influence asthma is not known. There is disagreement between experts over whether hormonal or antihormonal treatment is of any benefit. Some women do have life-threatening attacks premenstrually, with large drops in their peak expiratory flow readings. The problem may not improve much, even with high dose steroid treatment, but sometimes they do respond to progesterone hormone therapy, given by injection into the muscles.

Work

How do different working conditions (e.g. air conditioning, smoky rooms etc.) affect different people with asthma?

The type of work you do may be as important as your working conditions. Types of work which may affect asthma include working with particular animals, certain spices (mustard for example), dusts and fumes (for example, open gas fires and gas cookers).

Adequate ventilation at your place of work can help to reduce problems in all these cases. As far as working conditions are

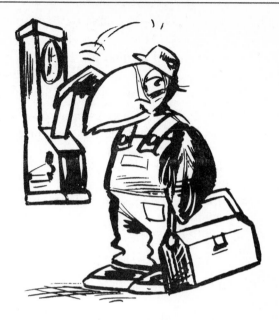

concerned, anything which pollutes the air may make asthma worse. Cigarette smoke is the biggest hazard. Air conditioning or heating may recirculate polluted air and increase problems rather than improve them. Fan air central heating may even cause spreading of virus infections (colds) which aggravate asthma. Many employers now realize the risk posed to the health of their employees by smoky environments, and they are banning or restricting smoking in the workplace. We welcome this, and hope it will become universal.

If you believe there may be a problem with your own work-place, discuss it with your occupational health service, if you have one, or possibly your union representative.

Are there occupations I will have to avoid?

Anyone with asthma should avoid occupations which are known either to cause asthma or make it worse. There are a number of occupations in the UK which are known to provoke asthma in previously healthy people. The Department of Health publishes a leaflet on these types of occupational asthma. The asthma may take anything from days to years to develop, and may not clear up when exposure to the substance that was responsible has ceased. People who have developed asthma after working with certain substances may be eligible for industrial compensation. Substances known to cause occupational asthma include:

- adhesives – in particular the isocyanates used in the manufacture of polyurethane, spray paints and surface lacquers – and epoxy resin hardening agents;
- animals and insects (laboratory workers and farmers);
- azodicarbonamide;
- drug manufacture – e.g. cimetidine and certain antibiotics;
- dyes such as carmine;
- flour, grain and coffee beans;
- ipecacuanha;
- ispaghula;
- metals – aluminium, cobalt, chrome, nickel, platinum salts and stainless steel;
- proteolytic enzymes – in baking, meat tenderizing and detergent manufacture;
- soldering flux (containing colophony or ammonium chloride);
- wood dusts, especially hardwoods (cabinet makers are more likely to develop occupational asthma than general builders).

There are other occupational causes of asthma. If you suspect that your work may be responsible for your asthma, you should consult your doctor to help you decide if you should be referred to an occupational specialist. This is important from the point of view of your treatment, compensation and future work.

Will asthma affect my son's future regarding employment?

With regard to employment, there is a small chance that a history of asthma may cause problems for young adults seeking work. However, people with asthma tend to be just as well qualified as those without, and therefore should stand an equal chance of being employed. Ill-informed employers who believe that they are anxious (or 'nervous') people are discriminating against them unfairly.

Certain occupations or conditions in the workplace could have a bad effect on your son's asthma. Any job which involves close contact with dust, sprays, fumes or poor air quality should be avoided wherever possible. Ideally, his workplace should also free of cigarette smoke. We realize it is not always easy to choose your workplace. If he gets a job with a large organization, he should be able to get help in improving his working environment from occupational health departments, or union representatives.

Will I be able to be a policeman?

There are potential difficulties for people with asthma who wish to join the Police Service, the Fire Service, the Armed Services or the Ambulance Services. We base the answer to this question on information obtained from the services in the London area. There may be regional differences in other parts of the UK and so it is worth contacting your local recruitment officers to check the information given here.

The Police Service will take advice from their medical advisers. Each case is assessed individually, so it is worth you applying. As a general rule though, they will not accept people who currently have asthma, or who have a history of severe asthma in the past. So if you had mild asthma in childhood there should be no problem.

The Army will not accept anyone who has asthma at the time of applying, or who has had the need for treatment in the previous four years. Any applicant who has been clear of asthma for four years will be assessed by the service specialist who makes the final decision. Anyone who fails to disclose important medical information may be dismissed from the service. It is worth bearing in mind that asthma may remit (go quiet for a number of years), but may come back at a later date. Someone joining the Army may be exposed to gases and other triggers which may make the asthma return. This is one reason why the Army is very cautious about asthma.

The Ambulance Service do not employ people with asthma. An ambulance paramedic may be exposed to air pollution and smoke when attending an incident, therefore it is very important to take preventer medication regularly if prescribed.

The Fire Service will not accept anyone with asthma for obvious reasons. Contact with smoke and noxious fumes is a necessary part of the job, and cannot be recommended for anyone with asthma, even if it is well controlled.

Holidays

Does travel cause any discomfort to people with asthma?

Travel should not normally cause any particular problems for people with asthma. However, any circumstances which cause a shortage of oxygen may be difficult. This may arise in common conditions such as flying in an aeroplane where smoking is permitted. Alternatively the reason may be more exotic, such as a holiday in the mountains at altitudes above 6000–7000 feet.

One of the biggest problems is that of being caught off guard if you have an attack when away from home. This is a much greater risk than that associated with the travel itself. If this happens while you are on holiday in the UK, and the symptoms are not severe, it is possible to register as a temporary resident with an NHS GP. It is the most suitable way to get help unless you are seriously ill. A GP will usually treat you more quickly than a casualty department, where accident and emergency cases are dealt with as a priority, and there are usually very long waits for people with emergency problems. All GPs deal with many people with asthma, and so will usually be experienced in the management of attacks. Accident and Emergency departments are really for emergencies. If you do need to be referred to hospital for severe asthma, then the local GP will know the arrangements for getting help more quickly from the local specialist. If, however, you suffer a severe attack it is wiser to go straight to hospital (see Chapter 6 on *Emergencies* for more about when to go straight to hospital).

If you are travelling abroad, the arrangements for emergency medical care are much more variable, and it is worth finding out about them before you travel. All travel companies and travel agents provide details on emergency medical arrangements for their clients.

Generally speaking, enjoy the journey! It shouldn't cause problems.

I am going on holiday, and don't want to take my inhaler with me. Is that all right?

No, it isn't! We assume you are taking both preventer and reliever inhalers, so let's look at them separately and we will try and give you reasons why you should take both of them on holiday with you.

It is essential that if your doctor has prescribed a preventer inhaler you should use it on a regular basis, even if you are fit and well and without asthma symptoms. It is by not using it that your asthma could deteriorate and go out of control, and your holiday could be ruined.

Your reliever inhaler is equally important to take with you, and should be carried with you all the time. You should really take an emergency pack for asthma attacks whenever you go away (see later question on precautions for children). Going to different parts of the country (or the world) can sometimes make your asthma worse even if it appears well controlled. If you don't have your reliever treatment at hand it could be very dangerous.

Will flying affect my inhalers?

Flying will not adversely affect your inhalers. It is better, though, that they are kept with you in the cabin rather than kept in the hold of the aircraft. It is important that your inhaler should be at room temperature when you use it – if it feels cold to the touch then warm it in your hands before use. Cold inhalers may not dispense the correct dose of drug. These comments only apply to pressurized canisters. Dry powder devices (such as Diskhalers, Accuhalers, Rotahalers and Turbohalers – Figures 2.1, 2.2, 2.8) are not affected by temperature. It is safe to use all forms of inhaler in modern aircraft.

My inhaler is pressurized. The airline regulations say that I cannot carry it in my luggage so what can I do? What if I need to use it during the flight?

Although the regulations may state this, airlines do recognize that people with asthma need to take pressurized inhalers with them on their travels. It is better and safer for you to carry your treatment with you in your hand luggage, in the cabin! Some airlines, including British Airways, carry their own emergency asthma treatment on some of their flights.

Can I get my usual inhaler in other countries?

Most asthma drugs are available in countries in western Europe, Canada, Australia and New Zealand with a doctor's prescription. The formulation, strength and brand name of the drug might vary slightly from country to country. Inhaled steroid treatments are very difficult to obtain in the USA. Also relatively new drugs such as Serevent, Foradil and Oxis and Oxivent may not be available yet in other countries.

Some of the newer inhaler devices may be more difficult to obtain than the traditional 'puffers' or aerosol inhalers which are now widely available throughout the world.

The medical information departments of the major pharmaceutical companies will be able to tell you which of their products are available in which countries and under what names. We would still advise you always to take an extra inhaler with you if you go abroad, in case you lose the one you are using. Also, take any necessary emergency treatment with you in case you have an acute asthma attack.

Will going skiing make it worse?

In our experience most people with asthma who take to the ski slopes have very few problems. If, however, your asthma is particularly triggered by cold air and exercise it may cause a problem. These days most ski resorts have an abundance of ski lifts so the struggle up the slopes need not therefore be particularly strenuous. A great advantage of going to a ski resort is that the house dust mite does not survive at 'snow' level so it is quite possible that, if the mite is normally one of your triggers, your asthma will be better when you are skiing than when you are at home. As with any holiday you plan to take, do make sure you make contingency treatment plans and know exactly what to do if an attack occurs. Do make sure also that you take out sufficient medical insurance cover, although this is usually compulsory in case of expensive skiing injuries, and so should be more than adequate!

If I do not normally suffer from 'exercise' asthma, will altitude affect me more than someone who doesn't have asthma?

The air temperature is often lower at high altitudes, and cold air may trigger asthma. The air is also thinner at high altitudes and there is less oxygen available. This affects everyone and may cause lightheadedness, nausea and swelling of the feet. This is well known as 'altitude sickness' or 'mountain sickness'. If your asthma is well controlled, you should be affected no more and no less than anyone else. Someone with severe or uncontrolled asthma would probably suffer more. On the plus side, the house dust mite cannot survive at high altitudes, and this is one of the main reasons why clear mountain air, as in the Alps, can be so beneficial for people with asthma.

If you are planning to go to high altitudes, i.e. above 5000 feet (this is well above the height at which most people go skiing), then you should take extra precautions to prevent attacks. Your asthma should be well controlled before you travel. If peak expiratory flow readings are not up to your usual best, it would probably be sensible to increase dosages until they are.

Once there, it is unwise to try and do a lot of strenuous exercise without giving your body a chance to get used to the change. It takes a number of weeks to become fully adapted to very high altitudes. Lightheadedness and nausea are signs of shortage of oxygen. Extra asthma medication and rest are advisable if this happens.

Will customs take away my medicines?

In most countries of the world there should be no problems about carrying routine medication with you. When you are travelling it may be helpful to take with you a letter or statement from your doctor confirming that any drugs you carry are prescribed for personal use. This does not guarantee that customs will not confiscate your medication. If you are in any doubts about the country you propose to visit, we suggest it would be safer to double check with the relevant embassy before you go.

What precautions should my young children take on school trips and holidays?

They should take enough medication to last for the time they are going to be away. They should be encouraged to take their medication regularly, and their teachers should be aware of the treatment. It would help to have a written treatment plan explaining the medication for the teachers' benefit.

Your children should know to call the teacher if they start getting symptoms (or if their peak flow rate starts to drop), especially if this happens at night. They should be reassured that there is no shame in calling for help if their asthma goes out of control.

For emergencies while away from home they, or the teacher, should carry a spare reliever inhaler (Ventolin Evohaler or Bricanyl), a short course of prednisolone tablets and a peak flow meter. A written emergency treatment plan helps to explain the use of these to the teacher, or adult in charge. All of this information can be written on one of the National Asthma Campaign's children's asthma cards. These are available to the medical profession and the public through the NAC. The address is given in the *Useful addresses* section of the Appendix.

Sports

Can I participate in any sporting activities?

If your asthma is well controlled you should certainly be able to play any sports, even if they are very energetic. It is important though that you receive, and take, the right treatment to prevent your symptoms from occurring. The majority of people with asthma should feel that they are not restricted in any way at all, in spite of their condition. There are many sportsmen and women who have asthma and it has not stopped them from representing their country or, for that matter, even becoming gold medallists!

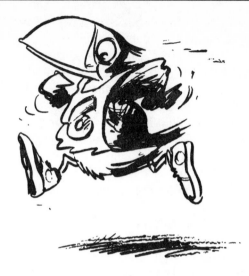

Paul Scholes, Karen Pickering and Jonathan Davies are three such stars who have asthma.

Is there any harm in doing regular exercise, or can this actually improve my asthma?

Regular exercise is good for everyone and providing that your asthma is well controlled it will certainly do you no harm. Studies carried out to try and find out if regular exercise improves asthma have only shown that overall fitness improves. Improved fitness results in improved lung function and improved wellbeing. This is not quite the same as 'improving asthma'. However, we have noticed from our own patients that many report that, if they do regular exercise, they get fewer problems with their asthma.

Why does swimming help people with asthma?

There are two main reasons for this. Firstly, exercise of any type helps to build up stamina and strength. Swimming does this for most of the muscles in the body, but in particular for those which help with breathing. Strengthening your breathing muscles helps to fight asthma attacks when they happen. Stronger breathing muscles also give you a better chance of controlling your breathing at times of difficulty.

Secondly, humidity in the air around a swimming pool helps counter the tendency to get asthma with physical exercise. Exercise in a warm moist atmosphere seems to be much less likely to cause symptoms than the same amount of effort given to exercising in cold dry air. It should be said, however, that the chlorine used to keep the pool clean may start off an asthma attack. If this is a problem it is probably wise to take a couple of puffs of your reliever inhaler before swimming to prevent symptoms.

The National Asthma Campaign has established many successful swim groups for young people with asthma throughout the UK.

Swimming is a sport that people with asthma can enjoy and in which they can have great success; this in turn can give them the confidence to participate in other sports. As long as their asthma is well controlled there is no reason why they should be restricted to swimming.

Isn't it dangerous to use my inhaler before exercise?

Quite the opposite is true. Using an inhaler before exercise is quite safe, and usually will prevent asthma attacks in those people whose asthma is triggered during or after exercise. Two types of inhaled drug are effective for this purpose. They are Intal (sodium cromoglycate) and the relievers such as Ventolin, Bricanyl and Airomir.

Intal is very effective as a pre-exercise treatment. In those people taking this drug, an extra dose can be taken about half an hour before exercise. The use of Intal in this way is permitted for competitive sports.

Ventolin and Bricanyl are reliever drugs. Everyone with asthma should have one of these with them at all times. They are usually used to treat and relieve symptoms of asthma. However, they may also be used at times when asthma symptoms are expected, such as when exercise is planned. Two puffs of the inhaler taken a few minutes before planned exercise is a very effective way of preventing problems.

Should I stop my child playing sport?

No! No! No! Some of our best known athletes and sports stars have asthma and you may be hiding a potential Olympic champion! It is a sad state of affairs but there are many children who have undiagnosed or uncontrolled asthma who give the appearance of disliking sporting activities. They frequently feel inadequate and 'wimpish', and compared with their schoolmates their sporting performance is poor. We often ask children with asthma what position they play on the football pitch, and 'goalkeeper' is the all too frequent answer. On closer questioning we find that they may have chosen to play in goal because the position does not require too much exertion, and it therefore prevents any ridicule from their team-mates. A good test of asthma control is to ask the question again after they have received good asthma care. Many times we have heard that after effective treatment they are able to play 'out' as well. It may be tempting for parents to stop their children from playing sport, and of course if the asthma is bad this is sensible because exercise can make matters worse. However, the aim should be for good asthma control with no limitations on activities.

Do remember, though, that on their own admission some children with asthma use their asthma to get out of having to do sporting activities even if it is not causing any problems at the time. Children with asthma are exactly the same as other children in that they don't all enjoy playing sport – the difference is that they can use it as an excuse for standing on the touchline.

Are there any sports that I should avoid taking part in?

The situation with scuba diving and asthma is not very clear. You will not be able to dive in the USA if you have asthma, but in the UK it is usually permitted providing your asthma is well controlled (no symptoms), with normal peak expiratory flow. You will need a medical certificate stating that your lung function is normal and your asthma is well controlled. We advise anyone with asthma, planning a diving holiday, to find out the rules in the country that they plan to visit.

Other sports that involve the use of pressurised air or oxygen, such as skydiving, might require caution, but you should take specialist advice on this. For the most part, assuming your asthma is well controlled, you should be able to participate in all other sporting activities.

I play football. Is it all right to take two more puffs at half time even though it's not four hours?

It is perfectly safe to take two puffs of a reliever earlier than four hours from the last dose. So, yes, it is all right to take extra relief medication during exercise. However, it is **not all right** to ignore the fact that, if you need to do this, your asthma is poorly controlled.

Regular preventive treatment should control asthma symptoms effectively. If this is not the case and you need reliever treatments frequently, as for example on the football field, then some adjustment to your regular treatment is required. Regular peak expiratory flow readings will help to show whether this is true or not. If the readings vary by more than 15% a day, from morning to evening, it is wise to consult your doctor or asthma nurse. It is very important to do this. Extra puffs of inhaler at half time should be a rare occurrence, not a regular one. If your asthma is better controlled, you will have more stamina on the field and your game should improve!

Becotide is a steroid – will my son be allowed to run in official sports?

As the Barcelona Olympics and the 1994 Football World Cup have highlighted, the use of drugs in competitive sport is a complicated issue! The International Olympic Committee (IOC) has taken steps to prevent drug use to improve the performance of athletes, but this has led to some confusion about certain drugs which are required for medical conditions.

Most asthma treatments are permitted but there are certain restrictions. The steroids used for treating asthma are in the group called corticosteroids, and are not the same as the anabolic steroids used to improve performance and increase muscle bulk. Your son will be allowed to use inhaled steroids such as Becotide,

Becloforte, Flixotide and Pulmicort. Anyone using corticosteroid tablets or injections at the time of an event will, however, be banned from competing.

Athletes with asthma are also allowed to use the inhaled relievers such as Ventolin, Bricanyl and Airomir. As with steroids, though, these drugs are not permitted in tablet or injection form. Another banned drug in sport is fenoterol (prescribed as Berotec or in Duovent).

Intal (sodium cromoglycate) and Tilade (nedocromil sodium) are permitted, as are aminophylline or theophylline drugs. Some brand names for these drugs are Phyllocontin, Theo-Dur, Slo-Phyllin, Nuelin and Uniphyllin.

Certain 'cold cures' may have substances in them that are not permitted. These include nasal decongestants containing adrenaline or isoprenaline, and any preparations with caffeine.

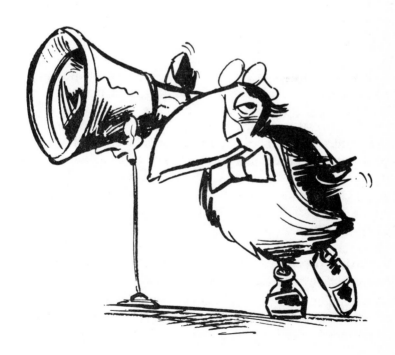

Pollution and weather

Are pollutants in the air causing asthma?

Outdoors, there are three major sources of pollutants in the air that we breathe.

1 Fumes from exhausts of motor vehicles which use petrol or diesel fuel.
2 Smoke produced from burning coal, wood and gas. Factories, industries and home coal fires are responsible for this form of pollution.
3 Ground level *ozone*, which is formed by a reaction between the sun's rays and other forms of pollution. Ozone is a gas, related to oxygen, which is found in small quantities in the air. This ground level ozone is harmful to the lungs, and our pollution is producing more of it. It helps to form what is called *photochemical smog*. Yet ozone in the upper atmosphere protects us against the harmful rays of the sun, and we are destroying it!

Indoor pollution is mainly due to tobacco smoke, perfumes, aerosol sprays and occasionally inefficient gas fires.

There is no doubt that these substances can make asthma worse and it is worth avoiding contact with them if at all possible. The problem, of course, is that we can have little control over the air that we breathe, except for tobacco smoke in the home.

The crucial question is whether increasing atmospheric pollution is actually **causing** asthma in previously healthy people. Many very polluted cities have low asthma prevalence! Research is going on at the moment, and the results will make the situation more clear. We hope future governments will take measures to improve air quality.

TV weather forecasters talk about poor quality air. Should I stay indoors or increase my treatment?

Poor air quality has recently been highlighted as a cause of worsening asthma control in certain individuals. As with people who are made worse by pollen, it can be very difficult to avoid this trigger factor. It may be sensible to stay indoors when there is very poor air quality, but in some urban areas this might effectively put you under house arrest for long stretches of the year! Probably the most practical action you can take is to step up your treatment during these periods. The amount and quality of information gathered about air pollution will improve greatly in the coming years, and we will all become much more aware of the day to day changes in our atmosphere.

How do atmospheric conditions affect people with asthma?

House dust mites are the most important atmospheric trigger factor for asthma. They probably do not qualify as 'atmospheric conditions', but they multiply during damp weather and they inhabit the air most often in the early winter months from October to December in the UK. Cold dry air in winter also tends to provoke asthma.

Thunderstorms seem to aggravate asthma in many people, so much so that hospitals are very busy during the day or two following a thunderstorm. The most likely explanation for this is that pollen gets released in these weather conditions. Therefore, if there is a storm, keep your windows closed and increase your dose of preventer medication for a few days.

However, there are important types of pollution in the atmosphere that may also make asthma worse. Some common substances are: car exhaust fumes; smoke from cigarettes, factories and fires; paint and glue fumes; and fog.

Ozone in the outer atmosphere protects people from harmful rays of the sun, but at ground level it is very irritant to the lungs. Ozone at ground level is increased by the reaction between the sun's rays and these types of air pollution.

All of these conditions can make asthma worse. Weather forecasts often include mention of levels of pollen, fog and other pollution as part of their broadcast. We need to be aware of how important these forms of pollution can be, and to agree how people with asthma can respond best to them.

My child was admitted to hospital with a bad asthma attack after a thunderstorm. Is this common?

There have been a few 'mini epidemics' of acute asthma during thunderstorms. During thunderstorms, pollen grains explode into tiny fragments small enough to be breathed into the lungs. Interestingly, asthma attacks following thunderstorms usually occur in people who have hay fever, and have never been diagnosed with asthma. As a result, these people don't have asthma inhalers and often end up in hospital when the attacks occur. People with hay fever who suffer from wheezing episodes are prone to future asthma attacks; they should consult their doctor for a prescription for a reliever inhaler for emergency use if needed.

Food and drink

Can I drink alcohol when I take asthma medication?

You can certainly drink alcohol when you take asthma medication, as none of the treatments should interact with alcohol. This is not, unfortunately, the end of the story! Alcoholic drinks can sometimes be a trigger for asthma. This may be caused by the alcohol itself, or the yeast, or preservative, or by other substances derived from the grain or fruit in the drink. It is not really known whether these reactions are allergic or chemical. Allergic reactions to yeast are common, and the yeast in beer which can trigger asthma in some people. The increase in home brewing has noticeably caused an increase in yeast allergy. Quite a number of people's asthma is triggered by wine. Some cannot tolerate vintage wines but have no problem with the cheaper varieties, while others are the reverse. We have known people who are aware that certain alcoholic drinks affect their asthma, but rather than avoid the particular drink in question, they increase their asthma medication before imbibing! Whilst we can understand this approach we cannot recommend it.

Why do I get asthma with red wine and not white wine?

Some people get asthma from drinking either red or white wine. Others, like you, are affected only by certain types of wine, or other alcoholic drinks. Some people get asthma just from drinking soft fizzy drinks. It just goes to prove what a variable and unpredictable condition asthma is!

As a rule, red wines contain more natural chemicals than whites. There is a particular type of chemical, aldehyde, related to alcohol which is found in red wine, and this may explain your problem. Many people find that red wine is more likely to give them hangovers, headaches or migraine, and these may also be due to this chemical.

Certain preservatives used in the manufacture of wine and soft drinks can start off an asthma attack. The commonest of these, at least in soft drinks, is sulphur dioxide (SO_2). If this substance appears on the label, don't buy the product!

I think my asthma could be due to a food allergy. I have heard about exclusion diets. What are they and should I go on one?

An exclusion diet is used in an attempt to discover whether any particular food or food additive is responsible for asthma symptoms. Such a diet should, in our view, only be undertaken under careful specialist medical supervision. There are two types.

In the first, any food which contains a suspect ingredient, for example egg, is excluded from the diet. Peak flow measurements are made twice daily for some days before starting the diet, continued during the diet, and after going back to normal eating. Usually the diet lasts between 10 days and three weeks. If peak flow measurements and symptoms become better when the food is stopped, and get worse again when going back to normal eating, the suspect food is responsible.

The second type of exclusion diet is used if no particular food is suspected, but it is felt that the asthma might be due to food allergy. In such a diet almost everything is excluded to begin with, except for only one or two foods. Lamb and pears are usually given as examples of the basic diet allowed, because they hardly ever seem to be allergens. One by one, foods are brought back into the diet. Peak flow measurements are again recorded regularly, and within a day or so of restarting the guilty food, a fall off in readings will be shown.

For both types of diet the whole process should be repeated twice to be absolutely sure that the changes in the asthma were not due to chance rather than the food. These diets can be difficult, time consuming and expensive. Foodstuffs are not very often important triggers of asthma, and so we repeat that we believe you need expert advice before launching into them.

Are certain foods unsuitable for people with asthma?

This is a fairly controversial issue. Some experts believe that asthma is never, or hardly ever, related to food allergy, while others believe that it is quite common. We feel that food allergy certainly exists, but that it is only rarely an important trigger for asthma. It is more likely to occur in people who have other allergic conditions, such as the skin allergy urticaria, and those whose asthma is triggered by, for example, dust, pollens and animals.

Sometimes asthma triggered by food allergy may take several hours to develop, and so food might not be identified as the cause. The most common food substances to cause asthma are cow's milk, nuts, soft fruit, shellfish, fish and yeast products. Food and drink additives can also cause asthma – see the answer to the next question for more details.

If you do identify a food or drink which definitely makes you wheezy, it is sensible to avoid it wherever possible. Failing that we recommend you take sufficient treatment to control your asthma and then to continue to eat what you want. It is important to remember that it is unlikely that food will be the only trigger, so regular asthma treatment may well be necessary anyway.

Are food additives bad for people with asthma?

Some of them can be. *Tartrazine* (E numbers 102–110 and 210–219) is the most common additive causing problems for people with asthma. This is a yellow colouring that used to be found in many sweets and soft drinks, although more and more often now it is being removed.

Food additives are marked on the labels of food containers in many countries, including the UK. We would advise that people with asthma should avoid tartrazine in particular. Other additives may also trigger asthma, but they may be very difficult to identify.

Sodium metabisulphate and sulphur dioxide (SO_2) are other examples often contained in fizzy drinks.

A peak flow diary may help in finding out if a particular additive is making asthma worse. The method for using this is explained in the section on *Peak flow monitoring* in Chapter 3.

Asthma and the NHS

I have to take asthma treatment regularly. Can I get any help paying for my prescriptions?

Needing asthma treatment regularly does not mean you qualify as exempt from prescription charges. However, at present, nearly three quarters of NHS patients do not pay any prescription charges. This is mainly because of their age, pregnancy or low income. If you are on income support you will be exempt from paying prescription charges. If you are on a low income you will need to fill in an AG1 form from the Department of Social Security and they will consider your application.

If, however, you are not exempt but do need frequent prescriptions, you can apply for pre-payment of your prescription charges (a *season ticket*) for a 4- or 12-month period. You will need to complete an FP95 form, available from Health Authorities, doctors' surgeries, some retail pharmacists and also the Department of Social Security. As this book goes to press, prescription charges are such that you will be better off buying a 4-month season ticket if you are likely to need more than five prescriptions during that period, or by buying a 12-month season ticket if you are likely to need more than 16 prescriptions over the year. (The season ticket will cover all your prescriptions, not just those for your asthma treatment.) However, by the time you read this, the figures may have changed, so be careful to check that it is worth your while before paying a lump sum in advance.

What is generic prescribing? Is this the same medicine?

Generic prescribing means that a doctor prescribes a drug by writing its generic name. Every drug has two names – its generic name and its brand name. The generic name is the name given to each drug when it is first developed. The brand name is the name given to the drug when it is manufactured by a particular drug company. So, for example, salbutamol is the generic name for both Ventolin, which is manufactured by Allen & Hanburys Ltd, and Aerolin which is made by 3M Health Care Ltd – these are both brand names. Pharmaceutical companies have to obtain a licence to start manufacturing a drug that hasn't originally been developed by them. They can then start producing it under a new and different brand name. Whilst all the drugs can have different packaging names, there are regulations to ensure that they all have the same constituents.

The advantage of generic prescribing is almost entirely that of cost. It is usually much cheaper to provide generic drugs than brand name drugs. Perhaps, not surprisingly, the disadvantage is that the cheaper, generic drug supplied may be of a lower quality. There are some safeguards to ensure the good quality of generic drugs in this country, but it is not unknown for cheap generic drugs to be imported from abroad and dispensed. In the UK about 45% of all drugs are prescribed generically. In asthma the proportion is lower than this, probably because doctors and those with asthma like to be sure of the quality, the colour and feel of the inhaler devices that they are prescribing.

My doctor says he feels my treatment is too expensive. What will happen?

We all have to be cost conscious these days, and there is no doubt that asthma is expensive for everyone. A conservative estimate puts the cost of asthma to the country at around £750 million per year, in terms of NHS costs, social security payments, and lost productivity at work.

Treating asthma costs the NHS about £400 million in total per year, and slightly more than half of this is spent on drug treatment. Correct treatment, even though it may seem expensive, costs less and is more effective (both for the individual's health and for NHS finances) than poor asthma control. It costs about £65 for one year's treatment for mild asthma at standard doses of beclamethasone. The costs for more severe asthma could reach £1000 per year.

In our view GPs should be encouraged to resist pressure to cut prescribing costs for asthma just for the sake of it. Instead they should concentrate on choosing whatever treatment is best for the individual patient. Good asthma management, including preventive treatment, not only makes people better and able to live normal lives, but can also cut NHS costs and days lost from work or school.

Those are our beliefs, but if your GP genuinely feels that your treatment is too expensive, you will need to discuss this carefully with him, and perhaps the Health Authority or Health Board. Your local Community Health Council represents your interests as a consumer of health care, and they may also be able to give you advice.

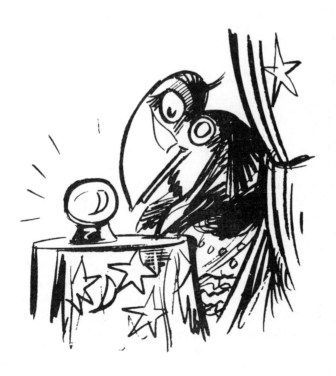

The long-term outlook

Does good control of symptoms make the long-term outlook better?

Good control of asthma reduces symptoms, making a person feel better. Very often people are unaware of how much they are tolerating in the way of symptoms, and if effective treatment removes these, then suddenly they feel dramatically better. Thus there is no doubt that 'quality of life' is improved by good control of symptoms. There is also good evidence that effective control of asthma symptoms reduces the number of acute attacks. These benefits are to do with short-term outcome of asthma, and what happens in the next few years. We cannot say for sure yet that the outcome in 15, 20 or 30 years will be improved by good asthma control. We believe that it is, but the research studies to prove or disprove it will take many years to complete.

In the meantime, we feel sure that the short- and medium-term benefits of good asthma control are sufficient to justify regular treatment, as long as it is effective.

As I get older, will it get worse?

This depends on how old you are when you ask this question! It used to be thought that nearly all children 'grew out of' their asthma by the end of their teens. Research has now shown that the outlook is not quite so good. Only about one in three lose their asthma completely. A further third either have a great reduction in symptoms, or their asthma stops only temporarily. The other third continue to suffer from asthma, although often in a milder form. In adults, the longer the asthma has been present, the more likely it is to have caused some permanent damage to the airways. In general, asthma does get worse as a person gets older, although even in adults asthma can improve or even disappear for many years.

There are other factors involved in getting older which may make asthma seem worse. Lung function decreases with age in everybody, so that we have less in reserve when we require extra air. Other conditions such as chronic bronchitis and emphysema also become more common with increasing age, increasing the problems posed by asthma. (See the section on **Related conditions** in Chapter 1 for more information about bronchitis and emphysema.)

The best way to avoid asthma becoming worse with age are to avoid smoking, to treat acute episodes early, and to take preventive treatment regularly.

Can adult asthma, like childhood asthma, be grown out of?

As we keep saying in this book, asthma is a very variable condition. It is certainly possible for asthma to disappear in adults, just as it does in children. However, you are far less likely to 'grow out' of adult asthma. People with late onset asthma tend to have continuous symptoms. It will certainly vary in severity from time to time, and maybe from season to season. It is less common for obvious triggers to be identified apart from upper respiratory tract infections (such as the common cold), which often make it much worse.

Sometimes late onset asthma can start because the patient has been prescribed a drug for another medical condition. Examples of this are aspirin, some of the anti-arthritis drugs (NSAIDs) and beta blockers (see the **Glossary** for more details about these groups of drugs). If this is so, and it is recognized quickly, stopping the drug can lead to a full recovery. In these few cases, one could perhaps say the asthma has been 'cured'. Similarly, patients who develop occupational asthma often improve when no longer exposed to the causative agent.

I am worried that my asthma could be affecting my heart. Could it do so?

If your asthma is well controlled you have no need to worry. People sometimes get palpitations after taking reliever treatment and worry that their heart is being damaged. This is not the case.

Uncontrolled asthma and severe asthma attacks may reduce the amount of oxygen that can be breathed into the lungs, and then transported in the bloodstream. This shortage of oxygen may put a strain on the heart, particularly if it is severe or if it continues for many hours or days. If there is a shortage of oxygen in the blood, the heart tries to overcome this by pumping faster and harder and the heart may get exhausted as a result of this extra work. In addition the heart muscle itself may suffer as a result of a shortage of oxygen. In practical terms this is rarely a problem, except in very severe attacks, or if the heart has already been weakened from some other problem.

Still, it emphasizes that it is very important to avoid severe attacks, and to try and maintain the best possible control of asthma for the rest of the time.

Regular exercise helps to keep the circulation in good condition. This enables the heart to increase its work when the person has an asthma attack. Smoking and other air pollutants interfere with the body's ability to carry oxygen in the bloodstream, and may put further strain on the heart.

Will I need to be on oxygen when I get older?

This is very unlikely, unless you have other severe chest problems such as chronic bronchitis or emphysema (see the section on *Related conditions* in Chapter 1 for more information about these). For such people lung function tends to become worse and worse as the years go by, and to have asthma as well may leave you very short of oxygen all of the time. Under these conditions oxygen in the home (domiciliary oxygen) may be needed. This is always best provided under the care of a hospital specialist in chest diseases. Modern equipment can extract oxygen from the air and concentrate it so there is no need to have great big oxygen cylinders cluttering up the front room. Also, the oxygen can be breathed through a small cannula (a soft plastic pipe) which fits neatly into the nose passages. This is much more comfortable than the old style of having a large mask clamped over the face for many hours a day.

Sometimes during severe acute attacks oxygen in high doses will be needed for a short time, but only to relieve the symptoms of the attack more rapidly.

5
Children and Asthma

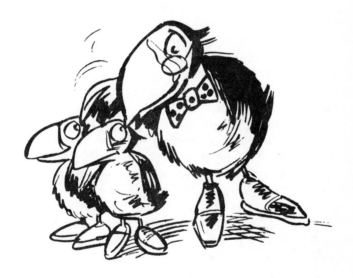

Introduction

Asthma is the most common chronic medical condition affecting children in the UK. Furthermore there is evidence to suggest that the proportion of children in the population who suffer from asthma is increasing. In the average primary school class in this country there will be two or three children who are diagnosed with asthma, and receiving treatment. Because asthma is now such a common condition in schools, much attention has been focused recently on problems faced by children in that environment. Many local authorities are establishing policies for looking after asthma in schools, and this should be a great advance. Until recent years many of these children were probably left undiagnosed. They were thought only to be 'chesty' or to have recurrent bronchitis. Now we appreciate how common asthma in childhood is, we can be more confident about making the diagnosis. Research has shown that, unless we do this, children go without the treatment they require to control their symptoms. As a result they lose much time from school, and miss out on a lot of social activities. So it is good to diagnose asthma when it is present, rather than hide it behind some vague term that nobody quite understands. The days when children with asthma were regarded as delicate, highly strung creatures should be well and truly behind us. Many of the questions in this chapter provide reassurance on the normal lifestyle that can – and should – be pursued by those children with asthma.

We also have sections on the two 'ends' of childhood – infancy and adolescence. Asthma in infancy is more difficult to treat, and poses a number of problems for doctors. Fortunately it is rarely severe. Asthma in infants probably varies widely, and these variants are the subject of much research at the present time. For example, one group of babies wheezes persistently for some time after a particular virus infection of the lungs called bronchiolitis. They may be troubled quite badly during infancy, but probably will not go on to have typical allergic asthma in later childhood.

For adolescents, it seems that problems are more frequent than we used to think. We used to believe that virtually all children lost their asthma during adolescence. Unfortunately this is not the case, and although many improve a great deal, only around one in three lose their asthma completely.

How and when does asthma start?

How young can asthma be identified?

Diagnosis of asthma may be difficult, particularly during the first year of life. Children under 4–5 years old cannot usually do a peak flow reading, which is the test used by doctors and nurses to prove their diagnosis. There is equipment in some specialist children's hospitals which can be used to prove asthma in young children, but this is not often needed, because a carefully taken medical history will usually provide the diagnosis. In very young children there are some clues to the diagnosis of asthma:

- children who cough a lot at night;
- children who cough a lot (i.e. need to see the doctor for this more than three times a year);
- children who wheeze from time to time;
- children who get colds which go onto the chest and take more than two weeks to get better;
- children who cough, wheeze or get chest tightness when they exercise or get excited.

A family history of asthma or allergy also helps in diagnosing asthma in a child who gets lots of chest symptoms. Where there are clues to asthma, doctors sometimes try a course of asthma medicines. If the symptoms improve (which may take up to eight weeks), this helps in making the diagnosis.

Our child has asthma – whose fault is it? There is no history of it in our family.

Without knowing the precise circumstances we cannot be sure, but it would be wrong to 'blame' somebody for the development of asthma in your child.

Most children with asthma have a family history of asthma, eczema or allergy (e.g. penicillin allergy or hay fever). These children inherit the asthma tendency in their genes. The asthma may only show itself when the child comes in contact with a trigger factor such as a cat, exercise, a cold or fog. Many children develop asthma even though no-one else in the family has it, but there will usually be some hay fever or eczema on one or other side of the family.

There is a connection between smoking and asthma. A child who is exposed to cigarette smoke in early life (while in the uterus and during the first few years after birth) is at greater risk of developing asthma. Therefore it would be wise for women to stop smoking before getting pregnant, and for parents to adopt a non-smoking policy in their home.

Is asthma more common in boys or girls?

Childhood asthma is undoubtedly more common in boys. In the UK it is somewhere between two and two and a half times more common in boys, although some surveys have suggested an even higher ratio. In most parts of the world asthma is also commoner in boys. The reasons for this difference are not clear. There do not seem to be any differences between boys and girls in the nature or severity of asthma. In adulthood men and women are affected in more or less equal numbers, and there is some evidence that late onset asthma is more common in women. Boys are more likely than girls to lose their asthma in adolescence, so this also helps to explain how the ratios come to be equal in adults.

Genetic studies suggest that the difference between boys and girls is not necessarily because of a difference in their genetic make up. There may be some other indirect factor, such as boys being more prone to respiratory infections than girls.

How can I find out how severe my son's asthma is?

It isn't easy for you to judge the severity of your son's asthma. This is particularly true if you have not had experience before of seeing other people with asthma. Another problem is that even people with mild occasional symptoms can sometimes develop severe asthma quite quickly. Not everyone fits neatly into a category of mild, moderate or severe asthma. We have to be prepared to accept that asthma may move from one category to another. You should talk to your doctor or asthma nurse, and they will be able to assess your son's condition. This is done not only by carrying out tests, but also by asking you carefully about your son's symptoms now and in the past. Asthma is such a changeable condition that it is important to keep a good eye on what has happened in the past, what is happening at present and to assess the situation constantly. Using a peak flow meter can help you to assess more accurately how severe any particular episode of asthma is.

Infants

When my daughter, 6 months old, coughs a lot, should I give her cough mixture together with the inhalers?

Most certainly not! There is really no point in giving cough mixtures to anyone with asthma. They are rarely of any benefit, and may even make matters worse.

- They may make the phlegm sticky, causing the air passages to become blocked. This can lead to a secondary infection in the lungs, which may require antibiotic treatment.
- They create a false sense of security. Parents may wrongly believe that they are treating their child and that no other treatment is needed. The asthma may get worse and the child may suffer unnecessarily.

It is safest to use the asthma medicines as advised by the doctor or nurse, and to call for help if this doesn't work.

Are those children who suffer croup in infancy more at risk of developing asthma?

No. Croup is a very unpleasant condition which causes narrowing of the larynx (voice box) and upper part of the trachea (windpipe). This results in a painful, barking cough and difficulty in breathing for infants and younger children. Like asthma episodes in this age group, croup is caused by respiratory virus infections (e.g. common cold). It often affects the same child repeatedly, but it is a separate condition, and does not put the child at any greater risk of developing asthma. There is another condition which infants get called *bronchiolitis*, and this does have a link with asthma later in childhood.

How do I strap my baby down if she is fighting away from the nebulizer mask or Nebuhaler?

It is a battle to persuade any breathless infant or child to take medication. When it is your own baby, it is even more difficult, but we hope you will not have to resort to strapping her down. Sometimes it is sufficient simply to hold the nebulizer mask a little distance away from the baby's face. If you hold it just below the level of her mouth then much of the mist will drift upwards towards her face, and be sucked in as she breathes. The small amounts which are breathed in by this method will be enough to give relief. Once the airways start to open, the baby often starts to relax more, and then will accept the mask. There are different types of face appliances with which you can experiment. Some babies are happier with masks, whereas others do much better with mouthpieces that do not need to be held over the face. There are other ways of approaching this problem. A Volumatic (Figure 2.10) or Nebuhaler (Figure 2.11) spacer device can be separated so that one open end is held in front of the baby's face. A large polystyrene cup with a hole cut in the bottom for the inhaler mouth is another version of this, and can be an excellent emergency method of getting reliever drug into young children (see Figure 2.14).

Will giving inhalers to a baby prevent asthma developing?

This is a difficult question to answer. It is not possible to tell which babies will develop asthma in the future, and as yet there is no case for giving anti-asthma treatment **before** the condition has developed. However, many professionals believe that **early, effective** treatment of asthma may well reduce the risks of any long-term problems. It may also shorten the duration of asthma symptoms. Evidence to support this belief is beginning to emerge, but it is still a controversial subject.

At present the main reason for prescribing inhaled treatment is to help reduce current symptoms and suffering due to asthma, and give a better quality of life. This is our practice, and we also believe that good control in the early stages of asthma means fewer problems in later life.

Perhaps we should also remind you that babies are not able to use ordinary inhalers!

Childhood

Is it safe to let my 8-year-old determine how much Ventolin to take when she is away from me?

Much depends on your child, and her attitude and capabilities. Perhaps the first and most important thing to remember is that, even if a child gets hold of a full Ventolin inhaler and takes all 200 doses, it will do them no harm apart from increasing their pulse rate for a short time, and making them feel trembly. This is reassuring but there are two other issues that need addressing: 8-year-old children can be very good at managing their own asthma, and can often stick to fairly simple guidelines. Most will be able to understand that they should take their Ventolin before exercise as a preventive measure, and also if they get symptoms. For these children it seems perfectly reasonable that they should be allowed to decide when to take the Ventolin.

The problems and dangers begin if their asthma gets bad, so that they require more and more Ventolin, but it ceases to be effective and they don't get help. This can be a particular problem if the child is using a metered dose inhaler, as it is impossible for anyone to know how many doses they have taken. The best way round this is probably for the child to take the Ventolin using a dry powder device. Ventodisks and Rotacaps are in single doses; the Turbohaler and Accuhaler are multi dose devices (the Accuhaler has its own counter) and the Ventodisks are numbered. She can be told that she may use a certain number of doses, and if more than that are needed then everyone will know that there is a problem. It is worth remembering that nowadays it is considered that relieving drugs (of which Ventolin is the best known) are best reserved for occasional use rather than to be used on a regular basis.

Could asthma cause my child not to grow properly because of his having constant poor health?

Uncontrolled asthma can certainly be responsible for poor growth in children. Growth hormone, which stimulates growth in the young body, is normally released in bursts during sleep and also during vigorous exercise. If your child does not sleep well or is unable to play sports then less of his growth hormone will be released. Also, children with severe asthma tend be underweight because they have much higher energy requirements than normal.

Atopic children in general, and children with asthma in particular, often have delayed puberty. This means they are often shorter than their friends in their early teens, but they have a prolonged growth phase in their late teens which may go on into their early twenties. Because of this, the eventual height of the individual usually reaches at least that predicted from their earlier growth performance; in other words, they usually catch up.

Is there any chance that I might give my child an overdose of the treatment?

The reliever drugs (Ventolin Evohaler or Bricanyl) are life-saving drugs when given in high doses. One dose of reliever from a nebulizer contains amounts of Ventolin Evohaler or Bricanyl equal to 15 to 30 puffs of the inhalers. These doses are safe, and we advise using them in an emergency. It follows then that it is unlikely that you can overdose your child with repeated doses from inhaler devices.

However, such repeated doses may be dangerous for another reason, and that is a failure to realize that this is a different attack, one that needs urgent medical help, and not just extra doses of reliever. In these situations, always seek medical advice, but continue to give the reliever inhaler while you are waiting.

It is possible to overdose people with the theophylline group of drugs (aminophylline, Nuelin, Slo-Phyllin). These should be used with caution and it may be necessary to have blood tests at times to make sure that the blood levels are not too high.

Inhaled steroids (preventers) have an upper dose limit, but this varies from person to person. Your doctor should give clear guidelines on your use of these drugs.

There are no risks of overdose with Intal or Tilade.

How old does a child have to be before he can be skin prick tested for allergies?

Skin prick tests can be carried out at any age, even on a new-born baby. They are painless when carried out by an experienced person. A negative test on the skin does not prove that a child does not react internally to an allergen. A positive test is a bit more helpful, in that it does confirm the presence of the allergic tendency (atopy). However, it can be wrong to conclude that the allergy in the skin is the same as the allergy in the lungs. The equipment for skin tests is imported from Denmark or the USA so currently most testing in this country takes place in specialist centres. However, it is possible that skin tests and simple blood tests for allergy will become available from your family doctor in the near future.

My child has asthma – how can I help make her lungs stronger?

Although it may seem surprising, your daughter's lungs are not necessarily any weaker than those of a child who does not have asthma. If asthma is controlled by giving the correct asthma medication to suppress the inflammation in the airways, the lungs will function absolutely normally. The best way for you to help your daughter to develop her whole body, as well as her lungs, is for you to encourage her to lead a full and active life with as few restrictions as possible. In this respect physical exercise is very important. Swimming is definitely one of the best activities to encourage physical development, and this is an ideal activity for a child with asthma.

In those few children with very severe asthma, special breathing exercises, taught by physiotherapists, may be necessary to improve the function of the lungs. Talk to your doctor if your daughter is in this group.

Can a child with asthma be underweight?

Children with severe or poorly controlled asthma are quite often underweight. Also, if there is a long delay in diagnosing asthma, children may be underweight and then improve considerably once treatment is started.

Recent detailed research has been carried out into the calorie intake needed for growth in children with asthma. It has been shown that they have greater energy (calorie) needs than children of the same age and weight who do not have asthma. This must be something to do with the extra effort required for day-to-day living with uncontrolled asthma. During acute asthma attacks, children may use up vast amounts of energy, and unless they make up for it quite quickly afterwards by eating well, they will lose weight.

Once the asthma is well controlled by the right treatment, the child can catch up rapidly in terms of weight and growth. We have all watched with pleasure such cases where underweight children with poorly controlled asthma have improved dramatically as their asthma has come under control.

In a similar way poorly controlled asthma may result in a child failing to gain height as well as weight. Although there are concerns that high doses of steroid treatment may affect growth, it is more often the asthma that retards growth rather than the treatment.

School

Should I tell a teacher that I have asthma?

Yes. It is important for your teachers to know about any problems you have which may interfere with your schooling. For example, in your science classes you may be working with substances that act as a trigger for your asthma. If your teachers know about this, they may be able to modify the experiments you are doing – perhaps simply by letting you use a fume cupboard so that you do not risk inhaling anything that could cause you symptoms.

Studies have shown that many teachers know little about asthma, but that nearly all are keen to find out more. If pupils can let their teachers know about how their asthma affects them, future problems may be prevented. PE is the single most important area of school life where the teacher should be well informed about asthma, and sensitive to the pupil's requirements. Unfortunately, our experience is that this is often not the case, and amongst secondary schoolchildren problems with PE are quite common.

The National Asthma Campaign (the address is in the *Useful addresses* section of the Appendix) has done a great deal to improve knowledge and management of asthma in schools. They have produced school packs, and also a school card which is completed by the doctor. This provides very helpful information for the teacher on the need for treatment. There are also guidelines on the action to be taken in an emergency.

My teachers don't like me to use my inhalers at school. Is it alright to miss my lunch-time dose?

It is important that your prescribed treatment should be taken exactly as directed. Many teachers do not realize the importance of regular preventive treatment for asthma and say that they find it disruptive to school routine if children need to use their inhalers. This is probably because their schools have a policy which requires that any medication needed by children must be locked away. For asthma, it would be far less disruptive if children had free access, or were allowed to keep the inhaler with them. It can be helpful if preventer treatment times can be built into the routine of the school day (for example, afternoon registration). Wherever possible, the reliever inhaler should be kept with you all the time.

Nowadays most of preventive treatments can be taken on a twice daily basis. In these cases your preventer inhaler can be kept at home, and need not cause a problem at school. It may be worth going back to your doctor's practice or hospital clinic to discuss your treatment, to see if twice daily doses are possible for you. If not, then it is important that you should have that dose in the middle of the day, rather than just forego it. Perhaps your parents, or your doctor, could speak to the school.

Can my son keep his inhaler with him in school?

As we have said in the answer to the previous question, some schools may have policies on whether or not children are allowed to keep their inhalers on them during school time. Unfortunately too many of them have such strict policies about all medicines being locked away that asthma treatments are often totally inaccessible. Even if your son is not allowed to keep his inhaler in his pocket, he should have free access to it at all times. Delay in taking reliever treatment can lead to a severe attack and could even prove fatal. Where possible, schools should involve the parents as to whether or not the inhalers are held by the pupil or by the school. For younger children it seems sensible that the inhalers should be kept by the teacher. For some older children at primary school, and for all those at secondary schools, the inhalers should be kept by the children themselves.

How can I convince other people (e.g. teachers) of the seriousness of my child's condition?

If possible, try and arrange a time when you can talk with your child's teacher without being disturbed. Unless you are absolutely sure of your facts, we suggest that you take some reading material on the subject of asthma with you – which you can then leave behind for the teacher to read. You could also take this opportunity to explain about the medication your child is taking and the importance of allowing free access to inhalers at school. It is also possible to arrange for a specially trained asthma nurse to go into the school to talk to all the school teachers about asthma. The National Asthma and Respiratory Training Centre has devised a special schools asthma teaching pack which is used by health professionals specifically for this purpose, and the National Asthma Campaign also produce an excellent schools information pack (see the *Useful addresses* of the Appendix for their addresses, and also see the answer to the next question).

Will teachers understand my son's asthma?

All the surveys carried out to date show that school teachers only have a very limited understanding of asthma and its management. Very few teachers have received any teaching or training about the condition. A survey testing the knowledge of school teachers in eight schools in London in 1990 looked at this. It revealed that whilst most teachers realized that asthma could be influenced by emotional factors, only one in three knew that taking asthma treatment before games could prevent asthma attacks.

Most of the teachers in the survey knew very little indeed about the various treatments, and unfortunately nearly half of them said they would not allow children with asthma to keep their inhalers with them. Some felt that children might overdose themselves, while others believed that children should be 'protected' from inhalers in case they developed an 'unhealthy attachment' to them!

Recently the National Asthma and Respiratory Training Centre (see the *Useful addresses* of the Appendix for their address), in conjunction with a group of school teachers from Gloucestershire, has been developing training material especially for school teachers. A very readable short manual has been written and a special teaching pack produced. These have been welcomed enthusiastically by the teachers. It seems that the chief problem in the past has been that teachers have felt poorly informed and ill equipped to cope with children who have asthma. This has often been seen by parents as a lack of interest by the teacher.

The National Asthma Campaign (see the *Useful addresses* of the Appendix for their address) have produced a Schools Asthma Policy Document. Schools can adopt and revise this to meet their own particular requirements. The document puts particular emphasis on the importance of preventing asthma symptoms – particularly in relation to sporting activities – and the necessity of providing easy access for the children to their inhalers at all times. It also gives guidance on what to do if a child has an asthma attack.

We feel that, at last, teachers are becoming far better informed about asthma. It will not be until all the teachers' colleges include training sessions on asthma, and all school teachers receive in-service training on the subject, that the situation will be ideal.

What if another child at school gets hold of my daughter's inhaler and uses it?

This is a common worry for parents because, rightly, they fear that drugs may be dangerous if given to the wrong person. We can assure you, however, that no harm would come to any child who used your daughter's inhaler – whatever treatment she takes. Children do sometimes use or play with metered dose inhalers that belong to children with asthma – they are wonderful for squirting at flies! Many a class room has had a liberal spraying from aerosol inhalers. This is far less likely to happen if a dry powder device is used, and we recommend changing the device to a dry powder one if you run up against this problem.

Growing out of it?

My 6-year-old son has asthma. Will he grow out of it?

This must be the question about asthma most frequently asked by parents and of course everyone wants the answer to be yes! It is very tempting when asked this question by a parent to say that all children will grow out of their asthma. Unfortunately this is not so, and obviously without knowing more about your son's medical history we cannot say what will happen to him for sure as he grows up. However, we do know that the milder the asthma the more likely it is that the symptoms will disappear before a child reaches puberty. Some children only appear to have their asthma symptoms (cough, wheeze and breathlessness) when they have an upper respiratory tract infection (a cold or sore throat). For them the outlook is good.

If, on the other hand, a child has asthma in association with hay fever and eczema, they are more likely to continue having asthma into adulthood. Strangely enough, the symptoms may often lessen or disappear at puberty even with these children, but they frequently come back later in adult life.

The earlier a child develops asthma, and the more frequent and severe their attacks, the less chance there is of the asthma disappearing in adolescence. As you can see, reaching puberty is even more important than usual for a child with asthma. By the age of 16 only 20–25% of youngsters will have persistent symptoms.

There are undoubtedly some adults who had asthma as children and then had no symptoms for many years (i.e. went into remission), only to find, in later life, that the condition returned. It is important to remember that once you have had asthma you are always going to have an 'asthma tendency' and the asthma can recur at any time.

Why did my asthma return? I had it as a child but then I was free of it for many years.

The simple answer is that we don't know. We do know that asthma sometimes returns after years of producing no symptoms at all. Most often this happens to young adults who apparently lost their asthma in late childhood. Most children with asthma first develop symptoms before the age of five, but most stop having symptoms by the time they reach puberty. By their late twenties, around 25% will have frequent asthma symptoms, around 30% will have no symptoms, and the remainder will be only mildly affected by their asthma. This is why we tend to talk about asthma going 'into remission' as young children grow, rather than being cured. We do not know exactly why this happens. The influence of body hormones at the beginning of puberty plays some part. In some cases, asthma returns in middle age or even later, as your question seems to indicate. This is even more of a mystery, though we feel sure there must be some trigger in the environment which can 'switch on' asthma that has lain dormant for many years.

Adolescents and young adults

I read somewhere that children who have asthma mature later than average. Why is this?

Research has shown that children with asthma tend to mature physically one to two years later than other children. The reason for this is not clear, but drug treatment does not seem to be the cause. X-rays of bones in children give a good indication of maturity. In children with asthma, *bone age* will often be one or two years behind the actual age. The practical effect of this is most important in adolescence, as they will have their growth spurt and their signs of puberty later than their friends who do not have asthma. Although we can reassure them strongly that they will catch up later, this may be of little comfort at a time when it is so important to them to be the same as everybody else.

So, in physical terms it is true, but there is no evidence that young people with asthma mature emotionally later than their peers.

I'm in the middle of my GCSEs, and my asthma has got much worse because of the pressure. I'm afraid that I might have an attack during one of my papers. How can I avoid this?

Early summer often brings problems for people with asthma. There are examinations, with lots of stress, but also the hay fever season with high pollen counts. Both of these make asthma worse in many young people. Prevention wherever possible is always better than cure, and there are a few things that may help.

April or May is a good time to visit your doctor or asthma nurse for extra advice on control of asthma. Regular peak expiratory flow readings kept on a record chart will be helpful in finding out whether your asthma is well controlled or not. If not, extra medication is needed, probably in the form of more preventer treatment. Medication for hay fever may also reduce the trigger effect of pollen on the asthma, even if you do not have the obvious hay fever symptoms of sneezing, running nose and itchy eyes.

Examinations bring on a lot of stress, and it is not easy to avoid this. Regular relaxation may help to reduce the chances of having an attack. There are many simple cassette tapes on relaxation available from pharmacists or health shops. This might be an activity the whole family can do together, and may help to reduce the overall stress that inevitably is around during this time.

If you are already in the middle of your exams, and your asthma is not under good control, make sure you carry a relief inhaler with you. Speak to your doctor about the possibility of a short course of steroid tablets to tide you over the most important days, although it is better not to be on oral medication during your papers if it can be avoided. If despite all this you do suffer badly through your exam time, a certificate from your doctor stating this may be helpful if the school or other people need to review your results.

6
Emergencies

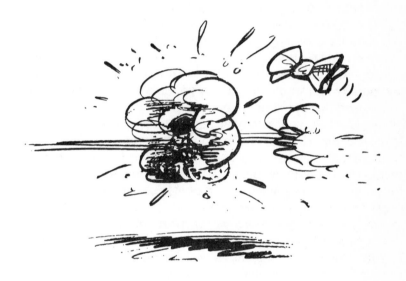

Introduction

In the last 30 years the number of hospital admissions for acute asthma has gone up dramatically in the UK. This rise has been particularly marked in children, most of all in the under-fives. The reasons for this are complex and have been the subject of much research and speculation. Whatever the reasons may be, there are now around 100 000 such admissions every year. Each one of these represents a failure of the preventive treatment which we are trying to promote. We have no doubts that, if health professionals and people with asthma could improve their recognition of the early warning signs of acute asthma, and take the right action, this number could be reduced considerably.

Throughout this book we have stressed the need to recognize uncontrolled asthma. This is because early action to remedy the problem is so important. The first section in this chapter deals with these symptoms and warnings. Probably the single most important sign is the failure of symptoms to respond to your usual reliever treatment. Don't accept this as just one of those things! It is a sign of potentially serious trouble.

The second section gives advice on what to do if an acute attack is upon you, or someone you are with. Although we work in the community and would like all our patients to stay out of hospital, we believe that for some people with asthma it is right to get to hospital as fast as possible during an acute episode. If this mean bypassing the GP, it should be done. However, one of the reasons for the enormous rise in hospital admissions for acute asthma is that perhaps too many people have taken this step. The decision to 'self-refer' to hospital is one that is best part of an agreed plan between hospital specialist, GP and the person with asthma (see the section on *Self-management plans* in Chapter 3).

The final section deals with recovery from attacks, which we feel to be just as important as early recognition. Everyone with asthma is more vulnerable to a repeat episode during the weeks following an attack, and it is a time when you should take very careful note of your symptoms and peak flow readings. Make a point of visiting your doctor or asthma clinic as soon as possible after an acute attack. If you have been admitted to hospital, clear arrangements for follow-up should be made before you go home.

First aid for emergencies

This information is given in more detail in the rest of this chapter, but for people with asthma and those around the essential points in dealing with acute asthma are as follows.

RECOGNIZE acute asthma, by worsening symptoms of cough, wheeze and shortness of breath, and failure to respond as usual to reliever treatment.

REMAIN CALM, encouraging the person with asthma to breathe as deeply and slowly as possible.

SUMMON MEDICAL HELP, either by calling the GP if easily available, or arrange transfer to hospital by ambulance WITH OXYGEN, if the attack is severe or there is difficulty contacting the GP.

CONTINUE TO GIVE INHALED RELIEVER TREATMENT until help arrives. There is no risk of overdose in doing this.

Symptoms and warnings

What are the warning signs and symptoms of an asthma attack?

Warning signs before asthma attacks vary from person to person. In one form, known as *brittle asthma*, people may go from no symptoms to severe acute asthma within minutes. For most people, however, there are warning signs before asthma attacks and these are of three types.

- Unusual symptoms which always or nearly always precede an attack. Examples of these are: a tickly cough; a strange sensation in the skin (usually an itch) or nose; lightheadedness or sickness. There are other warning symptoms and it is important for everyone to recognize their own.
- Your usual symptoms of asthma getting worse despite usual treatment.
- If you monitor your own peak expiratory flow, changes in the readings tend to take place before the symptoms start, and give

the earliest warnings of an attack. There are three patterns of change to watch out for:

1 steadily falling readings;
2 morning dips;
3 increased morning to evening gap in readings.

We have already discussed these changes in the section on *Peak flow monitoring* in Chapter 3.

The symptoms of an attack are the same as the symptoms of asthma – coughing, wheezing and difficulty in breathing. All of these may occur together, but during an acute attack shortness of breath is usually the most noticeable.

These symptoms should improve when extra relief medication is taken, and the improvement should last for at least four hours. If your symptoms are getting worse and do not improve with your usual asthma relief medication, or if they worsen again within four hours, then you should seek medical advice.

Asthma attacks come in varying severity ranging from mild to very severe. Mild attacks may only involve slight coughing, wheezing or difficulty in breathing. In a severe attack, there will be extreme difficulty in speaking and breathing. A person may become blue around the lips from shortage of oxygen (*cyanosis*). This colour can be very difficult to judge, particularly in artificial light.

A mild attack may develop into a very severe one. This may be sudden or take a few days or weeks to happen. It is for this reason that all asthma attacks should be taken seriously, even if they appear to be mild. Failure of relief medication to last for four hours or to have its usual effect is a very important sign.

'Everyone' seems to know how to treat an epileptic fit or diabetic emergency, but not how to treat someone having an asthma attack. Why? Is it the fault of first aid courses which give it such a low priority? Should there be more public education?

Asthma has had a very low profile until recent years, and very little attention has been paid to teaching people how to cope with someone having an attack. As it is one of the commonest medical conditions found in the developed world, there definitely should be more public education about it. First aid courses probably have given low priority to asthma, and we certainly hope this will change as public recognition of the importance of asthma increases.

There are good sources of educational material from the National Asthma Campaign and the National Asthma and Respiratory Training Centre (addresses in the *Useful addresses* section of the Appendix). In addition, the National Asthma and Respiratory Training Centre runs special courses for health professionals and also for school teachers.

Is it right that itching is a sign of an asthma attack?

Yes. Itching often comes before an attack, mainly in the upper half of the body. If this is one of your symptoms you will find that the itching tends to occur in the same area of the body each time. It is called 'prodromal itching' and occurs at an early stage of an asthma attack. It is usually something that children with asthma know about, although they may not complain about it. The cause is not understood, but it may be an allergic reaction. You can make use of this warning – if you take extra relief medication it may stop the attack.

If my chest feels very tight and my Ventolin is not working, what should I do?

As we have said many times in this book, failure to obtain relief from your usual reliever, whichever one you take, is an important sign of uncontrolled asthma. An attack may be on the way, and quick action is needed. Get medical advice as soon as possible. In the meantime self-treatment must be continued. Even though it may seem not to be working, it is important to persevere with your reliever in high doses until you can get other treatment. Ideally you should discuss with your doctor or asthma nurse what to do if this situation arises, but the following is general guidance. One puff every 10 seconds should be taken until there is some relief. If you have a spacer device available, take one puff every 10–15 seconds. This type of dosage is as effective as a nebulizer, and is perfectly safe when used as an emergency measure.

We would also recommend a dose of steroid tablets (prednisolone) at this time, if you have them available to you. A dose of between 30 and 60 milligrams for adults (6–12 tablets) and 20 and 30 milligrams (4–6 tablets) for children is suitable.

Once you have taken these steps, concentrate on breathing steadily, and staying relaxed until you can get further help.

What is a silent chest?

When someone has an asthma attack they have one or more of the common symptoms of asthma – coughing, wheezing and shortness of breath. As long as air is passing in and out of the lungs at a fair rate the wheezing will stay, and the breathing will tend to be quite noisy. However, when the air passages are so tight that very little air can get into the lungs there may be very few obvious symptoms. In particular there may be no wheezing, and in this case the breathing becomes very quiet. When a stethoscope is placed on the back no sounds of breathing are heard. This is described as a 'silent chest', and all doctors recognize it as a sign of a very severe attack. Emergency treatment is required for a silent chest.

Action to take

What is the best way for me to treat a very bad attack?

During a very bad attack it becomes difficult for you to speak because of breathlessness. This is an emergency which needs treatment in hospital. Take a high dose of relief medication: 15–30 puffs of reliever medication should be taken. This dose is **not** dangerous, but failure to take it might be. (It is approximately the same dose as that given in a nebulizer.) If you have a spacer device available, take one puff at a time every 10–15 seconds through this. Otherwise, use your device as best you can, repeatedly until you feel better. This is why it is important always to carry your reliever treatment with you. If possible take a peak expiratory flow reading and make a note of it.

Try to remain calm, and arrange to get to hospital. If your own doctor is with you he or she will arrange this, but otherwise call an ambulance if there is no one available to take you. Say that your asthma is severe, and that you need help urgently.

For a very bad attack a course of steroid tablets will be necessary, and if you have these available then the course should be started straight away. These tablets take approximately six hours to begin to work, and so it is important to start them promptly, particularly if you are away from home and there may be some delay in getting medical attention. Steroid tablets save lives in severe asthma attacks, and they should be used early in the attack rather than as a last resort. It is important to discuss this type of plan with your own doctor when you are well, so that you are more confident about what to do if you should have such a bad attack.

What is the best thing to do when I gasp for breath?

It may be difficult to stay calm when you are short of breath, but this is one of the best things you can do. Overbreathing as a result of panic will make an asthma attack worse. Relaxation exercises include practice at breathing slowly and regularly, and are good preparation for dealing with asthma attacks. Ask the doctor or nurse at your clinic for more information about these.

Having done this as best you can, take frequent doses of your reliever treatment, as described in the previous question, until you start to feel relief. If this is not effective, then you must seek urgent medical assistance.

Can I go straight to hospital if I have an attack?

Yes you can, and it may the best step for you to take if you suffer from sudden severe asthma attacks. If you are one of those few people whose asthma is bad enough to require several hospital admissions each year, then you will be under specialist care, and will usually have instructions on when it is best to go direct to the hospital. For most people with asthma this is not the case, and the majority of asthma attacks can be managed without the need for hospital admission. The general practitioner and asthma nurse are likely to be familiar with their patients' asthma, and in a good position to help deal with acute attacks. One recent national study showed that only one out of every seven people with acute attacks of asthma in the community were admitted to hospital.

How do we know when to take our child to hospital?

When asthma is diagnosed, whether in a child or adult, there are three questions which should be answered to your satisfaction by your doctor or asthma nurse.

- What should I do in an attack?
- How do I contact a doctor in an emergency?
- When should I go straight to the hospital?

If you haven't covered these questions with your doctor (or have forgotten the answers!) then go over them when you next have the opportunity.

In emergencies there are two possibilities. The first is to contact your general practitioner, and this is what we would suggest in most situations. It is usually best to see a doctor who knows you and your child's history. General practitioners in the NHS provide emergency cover 24 hours a day, although they have differing arrangements for providing it. Some provide it themselves, either as a practice or in a rota with other local practices. Others employ commercial deputising agencies to visit their patients after hours. (These agencies operate only in large towns and cities.) Your GP will be able to manage most asthma attacks without the need for hospital admission, but if admission is needed it is generally better for your GP to arrange this. However, if your GP cannot be contacted it is safer to go straight to hospital.

In other circumstances it may also be better to go straight to hospital. If your child has had a number of admissions to hospital for acute asthma, then it is desirable that a policy should be agreed with the specialist at the hospital. This is called an 'open door policy', and it means that, if your child has a bad attack which is not responding to an agreed treatment plan, you can take him or her direct to the hospital ward, without contacting your GP first. This is a sensible policy for children who have repeated admissions for asthma, and for adults with 'brittle asthma' whose attacks come on rapidly and can be very severe.

Most people do not have asthma that is severe enough to need this kind of arrangement, but it is much better for you to have guidance from your GP in advance of a problem, rather than afterwards.

Sometimes repeat doses of my reliever inhaler do not have any effect. What shall I do?

This is potentially serious! Failure to get a useful effect from repeat doses of a reliever is the most important sign of uncontrolled asthma. A short course of steroid tablets is probably needed. If you have a self-management plan that has been previously agreed with your doctor, then this should contain guidance on what to do. Otherwise you should get medical advice as soon as possible.

Can a child die of asthma?

Yes. Such tragedies are very rare but do occur. Of the 2000 deaths from asthma which occur each year in the UK, only 1–2% are in the under-14 age group (around 30 deaths per year). To put this into perspective, remember that 10–15% of children suffer from asthma, so that there are hundreds of thousands with the condition. Some asthma deaths are unavoidable. They result from sudden unexpected fatal attacks, nearly always against a background of very severe asthma or allergy (e.g. peanut allergy).

A fatal asthma attack in a previously healthy child is exceptionally rare. We would like to be completely reassuring on this point, but tragedies do happen, and so we must always be cautious if an attack of asthma seems different in some way from previous episodes, particularly if it responds poorly to reliever treatment.

What if I have an attack and I have no medication?

Ideally, this should never happen. Asthma attacks can occur without warning, and so you should always try to be sure that you have some relief medication available wherever you are. If, however, you have an attack and have no medication available, take steps to get treatment straight away, either from your GP or from the nearest hospital if your symptoms are severe. If the attack occurs when you are away from home in the UK, emergency treatment is available from any GP working in the National

Health Service. However, if you have a severe attack we would recommend hospital as the first choice. If you are in doubt about how severe your attack is (and it can be difficult), always err on the side of caution and go to a hospital.

If you are abroad without medication we would advise you to go directly to hospital if possible. In an untreated attack, delay can be serious, and on some occasions has been fatal.

What do I do if I am with someone having an asthma attack?

Stay calm. This may seem obvious advice but it is very important. Ask the person having the attack if they have their reliever inhaler (Ventolin or Bricanyl) with them. If they have, help them to take large doses of the inhaler as best they can. For an aerosol spray, this can be done by making an emergency spacer device using a piece of paper rolled into a cone, or by making a hole in the bottom of a paper or plastic coffee cup (see Figure 2.14). Hold the cone in front of the face, and fire the inhaler every 10 seconds or so, so that he or she can breathe the spray via the cone or cup. It is safe to give 15–30 puffs in this way, and this will nearly always bring some temporary relief. For the dry powder devices this cannot be done, but you can give repeated doses without risk of overdose.

While you are giving this treatment, arrange for someone to call an ambulance if the attack is severe.

Is it necessary to consult a doctor before administering Ventolin nebulizer to a person with asthma?

This treatment may be lifesaving in a severe attack. Since there are no dangers from using a **single** dose in this way, it is probably better that you start treatment immediately and then call the doctor for advice.

The potential problem in doing this does not come from the nebulizer, or even from the drug in the nebulizer. The danger comes from not recognizing when asthma is getting worse. If someone needs a nebulizer for an attack, it must be understood that the asthma is out of control. If the nebulizer relieves the symptoms for at least four hours, then the attack has responded to the treatment, and you should continue with your treatment plan.

However, if this does not happen, it is important that other treatment should be obtained.

We would advise that a short course of steroid tablets is also needed whenever an attack is bad enough to need treatment with a nebulizer. By all means give the nebulizer if it is needed, but contact the doctor for advice at the same time.

My sister has asthma. How can I help her if she starts to hyperventilate?

Hyperventilation (or overbreathing) means breathing more rapidly than is necessary or than is good for you. It occurs commonly in people who are anxious or frightened (whatever the reason), and causes symptoms of light-headedness, feeling sick, and tingling in the hands and feet. For someone with an asthma attack, who is trying desperately to breathe, it is an understandable reaction. Anything which helps to slow down her breathing will help your sister, including a gentle and calm approach by those around her. Extra use of her reliever medication will help to improve the asthma attack and this, hopefully, should reduce her hyperventilation.

The well known trick of breathing in and out of a paper bag is less helpful in asthma than in other circumstances. There is already a shortage of oxygen, and this may be made worse by breathing in used air from a bag. It will be more useful to talk slowly and reassuringly to your sister in order to slow down her rate of breathing.

How bad does an attack have to be before seeking medical advice?

Everyone's asthma is different, and so the detailed answer to this question depends a great deal on the features of your own asthma. Past experience is often helpful in deciding whether you need help. Ideally you and everyone else should have a self-management plan for treating asthma episodes (there is a section on *Self-management plans* in Chapter 3). When your asthma goes out of control, you follow the plan. If your symptoms fail to improve it is a sign that you need medical advice. Severe symptoms mean you must call for medical help straight away. Such symptoms are:

- difficulty in speaking, or being unable to complete sentences in one breath;
- severe difficulty in breathing;
- blue discoloration of the lips or tongue;
- very fast pulse (more than 120 per minute in an adult or more than 140 per minute in a child);
- very fast breathing rate (more than 25 per minute in an adult or more than 40 in children aged 5–15 years and more than 50 per minute in preschool children);
- becoming exhausted by the attack;
- peak flow reading less than half the usual level.

If you are unsure, it is always better and safer to seek advice early in an asthma attack, rather than later. The worse your asthma attack when you ask for help, the more difficult it is to treat.

Recovery

Why am I always sick after an asthma attack?

The sickness may be part of the attack, as vomiting is a symptom of asthma in some people. These people develop sickness as one of their early symptoms of attacks, and the vomit often contains a lot of mucus or slimy liquid. The attack may be mild to severe and sometimes causes a severe loss of fluid (dehydration) with the need for hospital admission. Because this symptom is uncommon the diagnosis of asthma may be delayed. The clues to diagnosing asthma are usually present at the end of the attack, when the vomiting lessens. The more common symptoms of shortness of breath and wheezing tend to be present at this stage.

Oxygen shortage during attacks is another possible explanation for vomiting. Asthma attacks cause narrowing of the airways, which means air can't get through to the lungs very easily. This can cause a shortage of oxygen in the blood, which may result in a feeling of sickness. A similar thing happens when people (with or without asthma) go up to high altitudes and develop 'altitude' or 'mountain' sickness.

For how long do I need to continue a higher dose of my inhalers after I have had a cold?

This is another of those situations where individuals vary, and there is no figure, or time, that applies to everybody. No one knows the right answer. You are doing the right thing by increasing your medication when an important trigger factor, such as a cold, comes along. The trigger makes the airways hyper-reactive or twitchy, and this may lead to a bad attack of asthma. It is wise to try and prevent this by increasing the use of relief medication as well as the preventer (if you usually take both of these).

One simple plan is to double your preventer dosage, and to take extra relief medication for symptoms as necessary. The increased dose should be continued until your asthma is stable again. This may be judged either from your symptoms or from your peak flow chart. When your symptoms have cleared up, the twitchiness of

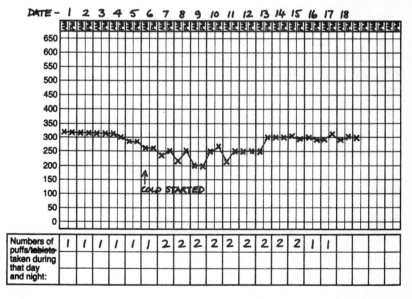

Figure 6.1 A chart showing how a child's peak flows dropped during a cold. This was treated by the family by doubling the dose of inhaled steroid (preventer).

the air passages has probably settled. A rule of thumb is to continue on the higher dose for two weeks after this time. Then the dose of preventer can be reduced to your previous level. This method often works well.

A peak flow chart gives a more accurate picture of when the asthma episode is over. Figure 6.1 shows a peak flow chart of a boy whose asthma went out of control due to a cold. It is clear from the chart when his asthma returned to normal. The peak flow chart method is best because it helps in two ways. It ensures that you take enough extra medication, because the dose can be increased until the readings settle. Secondly, once your readings have settled, you can reduce the dose. This means that you do not take more medication than you need (see Figure 3.9).

Normally your readings should be about the same whenever they are taken, but if your airways are twitchy, they will vary greatly from morning to evening (see Figures 1.5, 3.6 and 3.9). Once your readings have settled down and are back to normal, the dose can be reduced to your usual level. The continued use of your chart will then help you to decide whether this dose is sufficient.

We go into more detail about how you can use your chart to work out when it is safe to reduce your dose to its normal level in the section on *Self-management plans* in Chapter 3.

7
Non-medical treatments for asthma

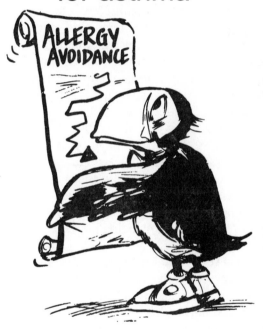

Introduction

This chapter is in two sections, but both are about the possibilities of treating asthma without drugs. We are not fond of prescribing drugs for the sake of it, but we do so because they are effective and have been shown to work in carefully controlled medical research. Any drug may cause side effects in a minority of people, and because of this we fully understand why many people wish to explore the possibilities of non-drug treatments for their asthma (or, especially, for their children's asthma). However, the benefits of drug treatment for asthma usually greatly outweigh the potential disadvantages from side effects.

Our difficulty is that very few of the non-drug treatments for asthma have been shown to be effective in true research studies. We feel anxious about patients stopping treatments that have been proved to work, in favour of treatments which **might** work. Uncontrolled asthma can be dangerous. This is why we would prefer such treatments to be *complementary* rather than *alternative*. By complementary we mean that they can be taken or tried alongside your conventional treatment. If they are effective – and sometimes they will be – then your asthma will improve and you will be able to reduce your usual drug treatment gradually. To stop effective drug treatment abruptly is potentially dangerous, and we would not recommend it.

Doctors are sometimes accused of being 'anti' complementary treatments for the sake of it. We have open minds about most of them, but we require convincing evidence of their effectiveness before considering them as first-line treatments for asthma.

The second section of this chapter deals with allergen avoidance. This is a particularly topical issue for two reasons. Firstly, a wide range of products is now being marketed, all of which make great claims for improving asthma by getting rid of allergens (mainly the house dust mite) from the home environment. Some of them may be very effective in reducing mite numbers but not necessarily symptoms. Nearly all are expensive, so we recommend you get specialist advice before spending too much money in the hope of a miracle cure. Having said this, exciting research evidence is beginning to appear concerning the possibilities of reducing the severity of asthma, or even avoiding it, by keeping babies away from allergens during the important first few months of life. There are no questions which directly address this topic, but research studies are taking place, and we hope that encouraging results may soon be available.

We should all be concerned to keep the use of drugs for asthma down to the minimum necessary. This chapter reflects those concerns, but we do believe that there are as yet no alternative or complementary treatments which are as effective as the preventers and relievers described in Chapter 2.

Complementary therapies

Do you think that complementary medicine can help people with asthma?

Yes, we do. However, there is little scientific evidence that these treatments used **on their own** are effective. They can be of help in some people when used together with the conventional medical treatments. It is better to view them as 'complementary', rather than alternative. The idea of treating the whole person, rather than the illness, is an important part of many complementary therapies, and one which we strongly support.

There are several complementary treatments available (see the next question), but we want to stress that the use of any of them should be in **addition to** and not instead of the conventional medical treatment. There is no place for these treatments in the management of acute asthma attacks, which are potentially dangerous.

What complementary therapies are available? Are there any ethical problems with the use of these?

There are three forms of complementary therapy which we believe may be of value in chronic asthma, as there is some research evidence for their value. We recommend that usual medical treatment is continued alongside these treatments, at least until they have started to give benefit. These disciplines are acupuncture, yoga and hypnosis.

Hypnosis may help by improving relaxation. However, there is a risk that under these circumstances important symptoms may not be recognized. This may be dangerous and so, if you try hypnosis, we would advise regular use of a peak flow meter to help identify whether your asthma is remaining well controlled.

Osteopathy may help to improve muscle spasm in the chest wall, which may help to make the breathing easier. Therefore this form of treatment may be worth trying in addition to usual medical treatment.

There is no scientific evidence that naturopathy, aromatherapy or reflexology are of help to people with asthma. The methods of hair analysis and iridology for diagnosing allergy and asthma have not been proved and are often misleading.

Does homeopathic treatment help asthma or make it worse?

Some research has shown that homeopathy may help people with hay fever. The situation with asthma is unclear as there is not enough good scientific evidence for us to be sure.

It is usual to test treatments claimed to be of benefit by doing clinical trials. These are research studies which compare the treatment in a number of groups of patients. The research is done by giving the test drug (the one claimed to help) to some patients while another group of patients is given a 'dummy' drug, called a placebo. The placebo drug is made up to look and taste the same as the one being tested. These studies are done in such a way that neither the doctor nor the patient knows if they are using the placebo or the real drug. Homeopathy has been tested scientifi- cally in this way more often than many other complementary therapies. None of the trials has shown that it is helpful in asthma, but on the other hand there is certainly no evidence to suggest that it makes asthma worse. However, if usual treatment is stopped when the homeopathic treatment is started, the asthma may deteriorate. This is why we advise strongly that usual asthma treatments should be continued when a complementary therapy is first tried.

Are breathing exercises and relaxation beneficial? If so, why are they never recommended by doctors?

Nowadays most doctors feel there is only a limited place for breathing exercises for people with asthma. Generally, they are useful only for those people with the most severe asthma. During an asthma attack the muscles around the airways tighten up, and the most important thing is to get these muscles to relax and open up the airways. We have no conscious control over these muscles, and the best way to relax them quickly is by giving reliever treatment. Fortunately this is usually very effective and works rapidly.

Although breathing exercises are not often recommended, general relaxation exercises and **controlled** breathing can be extremely helpful. When an asthma attack begins, it is easy for someone to become distressed, and to overbreathe (hyperventilate). In the panic of an attack, your breathing becomes rapid and shallow. This can irritate your airways and actually make matters worse. It is very helpful to learn how to breathe in a slow, relaxed way to prevent it from happening. You should practise this in between attacks, when you are free of symptoms.

Allergen avoidance

My asthma is due to house dust. Would one of the air purifiers or ionizers available on the market help?

There is controversy over how useful removing or reducing the levels of house dust and house dust mite in the home is. It is particularly in the bedroom that the problem needs to be addressed. There are now many preparations and devices available which claim to reduce dust levels, kill off the mites or purify the air. Unfortunately, for most of them, there is still no good scientific evidence that they are effective in reducing asthma symptoms. This applies to air purifiers.

The air contains many tiny particles which carry an electric charge, positive or negative. Ionizers are machines which change positively charged particles in the air to negative, and this has the effect of removing them from the air. One research study found that, by this action, an ionizer reduced the amount of house dust mite in the air in children's bedrooms. However, there was no improvement shown in the children's symptoms. Instead another research survey showed that they were in fact made worse!

If you are thinking of buying one of these expensive devices we suggest you contact the National Asthma Campaign (address in the *Useful addresses* section of the Appendix) for the latest information on their benefits.

Is asthma aggravated by using a vacuum cleaner? If so, there are some very expensive vacuum cleaners which claim to alleviate this problem. Are they effective?

House dust and house dust mites are found in huge quantities in all carpets, though less so in those made from synthetic fibres. Often vacuuming leads to a large increase in the amounts of dust in the air, and so does actually make asthma worse. Some preparations, including carpet shampoos, will kill off house dust mites, but this in itself will not do much to help. Some powerful vacuum cleaners will go a step further by removing much of the dust and the dead mites from the carpet. However, it is the amount of dust and house dust mite allergen in the air (and in the bed mattress) that is more important. **We are not convinced that the use of these expensive vacuum cleaners is of benefit in asthma.** Better results are more likely to come from reducing dust and mites in the bedding.

Should we have the cat put to sleep?

Once asthma has developed in response to a trigger (e.g. a cat, feathers, house dust mite etc.), it tends to persist for some time, even after removal of that trigger. So removal of a cat or any other pet from the home may not cure the asthma instantly. It is also the case that once one trigger has started off the asthma, other triggers may become equally important in maintaining the condition. Removing a much loved family pet sometimes causes so much upset that asthma may become worse for a while. On the other hand, there is some evidence that asthma can improve after removing a pet from the home. Fur or hair from pets helps the house dust mite to grow. Reducing the house dust mite numbers by getting rid of pets may help to explain this finding. Washing or wiping the cat with a damp cloth once a week may reduce allergy problems, but this is easier said than done!

As you may guess from this answer, having the cat put to sleep is not a simple solution to the problem of asthma, even if you or your child have a true allergy to cats. We recommend that you discuss the question carefully with your doctor, and in any case see if you can find an alternative home for your pet before having the poor cat put to sleep.

Is it a good idea to experiment with desensitizing treatments for specific allergies, e.g. to cats?

Not as a general rule. There are a few circumstances under which a specialist might advise this. Our general advice is that it is much safer to try and avoid substances or animals that trigger asthma attacks. Desensitization involves injecting you with tiny amounts of the substance (e.g. grass pollen) to which you are allergic. This enables your body to build up a resistance to the allergen over the period of time for which the injections are given. Treatment usually lasts for several weeks or months and, if it is successful, will be effective for years. The problem is that the injections may have serious complications. There is a risk of provoking asthma, collapse and even death. Serious reactions are uncommon. However, this form of treatment is much less frequent now than in the past, and is only available in specialist centres.

Desensitization is reserved for those unfortunate people whose lives are at risk from allergy to a substance. An example of this is bee sting allergy, which can be dramatically severe. It is not possible completely to avoid the risk of contact with bees and so desensitization is an important treatment option.

Conventional mattresses obviously harbour the house dust mites. Are there any materials which are better for mattress construction?

Not for mattress construction, but there are some mattress covering materials being used in experiments in asthma treatment. The idea is to cover the mattress with a material which does not allow the mites to penetrate and occupy the mattress in great numbers. Polythene or plastic coverings will do this, but they tend to make the mattress hot and uncomfortable, and can be noisy whenever you roll over in bed. This can be annoying, particularly if sleep is already difficult because of asthma!

There are new materials available which have pores that are too small for the mite to penetrate, but large enough for air to circulate to the mattress (see the *Manufacturers* Appendix for addresses). Research has shown that the use of these covers can reduce the symptoms of dust-induced asthma considerably. However, they are very expensive! But they may be worth you considering if your asthma is noticeably related to dust allergy.

Should I buy a mattress cover for my daughter's bed?

If your daughter's asthma is noticeably related to dust allergy, especially the house dust mite, it may be worth trying. We have discussed the type of cover in the previous question, but there is no guarantee that it will help. If you do decide to buy a mattress cover it should completely cover the mattress with allergen proof casing and the seal should be covered with tape. Remember, too, that you will need to have a special cover for the pillow case and also for the duvet. (Special mattress covers and pillow cases can now be purchased from large stores.) Avoid a padded fabric headboard. Even these measures will not remove all the mites from the bedroom.

The issue of reducing house dust mite numbers in bedrooms is a very important one, but it is not an easy task to carry out.

What sort of carpet is best for my child's bedroom?

The debate here is similar to that in the previous question. Not all children have asthma which is triggered by allergy to house dust and house dust mite. If, for example, your child's asthma is triggered by virus infections or exercise, then the type of carpet in the bedroom will not make much difference to the asthma. But if your child's asthma is clearly related to allergy, then the choice of bedroom floor covering can be important. Hardwood or linoleum floors are actually preferable to carpet because they cannot harbour dust in the same way. If a carpet is needed, then it would be better for you to choose one that is tightly woven and made of synthetic fibre. The house dust mite, which is the chief culprit, prefers to live in natural, rather than artificial fibres.

It is also worth remembering this when choosing curtain material, blankets, sheets and also cuddly toys. Whenever possible all soft furnishings should be washed frequently as this will cut down on the army of dust mites.

It is worth noting that it is allergen levels in the air that cause problems, rather than allergen levels in the carpet. However, if carpet levels can be made very low, then air levels will also fall.

I am told that the house dust mite likes soft toys. Is there anything I can do to reduce the number of mites on the toys?

There are many general measures which may be taken to reduce the overall numbers of house dust mite in the home. There are some new methods available, and some new preparations, called acaricides, which kill house dust mites very effectively. However, there is much research still to be done before we can recommend using these methods, which take time and money to perform properly, and may or may not be useful.

There is one rather unusual, but cheap and effective, way of reducing mite numbers on soft toys. We recommend that you put them in the freezer for at least six hours a week, and then vacuum clean them. This will exterminate the mites!

8

Self-help for asthma

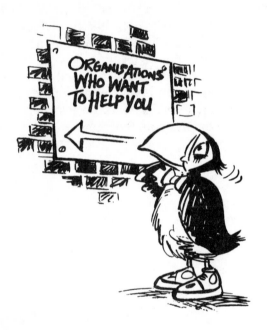

Introduction

We hope we have written enough in this book to convince you that
we believe the role of the person with asthma in managing their
condition is more important than that of the doctor or nurse who
advises on treatment. Self-help groups for people with all sorts of
medical problems have mushroomed in recent years, partly
because of a wish for mutual support, but also in recognition of
the way in which they wish to play a much more active role in

management of their condition, and in support of research. Asthma is no exception to this trend. The Asthma Research Council was established more than 60 years ago, and over the years has contributed enormously to the funding of important research into asthma. In 1980 the Asthma Society and Friends of the Asthma Research Council was formed, establishing a network of branches across the country. In 1990, these two charities merged to form the National Asthma Campaign. This is now the largest charity working solely for asthma, and gives more than £2.5 million each year to research. There are other charities giving tremendous support to research into asthma.

Only a small proportion of those with asthma are involved in any way with self-help groups. Many people feel that they focus too much attention on asthma, rather than encouraging a positive attitude to ignore it, and carry on regardless. We have some sympathy, but disagree. The asthma charities' aim is to help people live their lives fully, with minimum interference from their condition. We urge anyone with asthma to support the asthma charities in their work as much as possible, even if this is only from a distance in the form of a small annual subscription. Addresses of the charities are given in the *Useful addresses* section of the Appendix.

Asthma charities

Is there an asthma charity and, if so, how can people help?

The main asthma charity in the UK is the National Asthma Campaign. It was formed in 1990 by the merger of two smaller charities – the Asthma Research Council, and the Asthma Society and Friends of the Asthma Research Council. The much larger single charity has been very successful and has raised millions of pounds for research and education. You can help by joining as a member (an application form is provided in the back of this book) and by contributing and helping at a local branch of the Campaign.

There are two other charities which raise large sums of money for research into asthma: the British Lung Foundation was formed in 1987, and supports sufferers of all kinds of lung disorders and conditions; and the Chest, Heart and Stroke Association in Scotland and Northern Ireland has a long tradition of supporting patients with chest illness.

Are there any groups where I can get sympathy and understanding?

We suggest you join a local branch of the National Asthma Campaign. There are around 90 branches throughout the country. Each branch has members with a wide experience of asthma and the practical problems that can be associated with it. They can provide you with a lot of information and support which you in turn may be able to pass on to other people with asthma. The National Asthma Campaign also provides an Asthma Helpline run by specially trained nurses. This is open from 9.00am to 7.00pm from Monday to Friday (telephone number (0845) 701 0203, calls are charged at local rates).

In addition, some general practices have special times set aside for people with asthma to meet together, and to be able to ask advice from an asthma nurse or the general practitioner.

Information about asthma

Is there a video about asthma I can understand?

Many people find videos about asthma more useful and interesting than books or leaflets. The National Asthma Campaign has a range of informational videos which have been made for patients, including some for ethnic minorities. These are most easily viewed at branch meetings, but the Asthma Helpline (details in the previous question) may also be able to provide details. Several pharmaceutical companies also produce videos for patients that are very helpful but not always easy to obtain. It is worth writing to enquire about availability (addresses are in the section *Manufacturers* in the Appendix).

Is there any literature available which is easy to understand?

Yes. The National Asthma Campaign has an excellent series of leaflets which are constantly being updated. Similarly many pharmaceutical companies produce excellent booklets for adults and children. Nearly all general practitioners' surgeries, pharmacists and hospital outpatient departments hold stocks of a wide range of these leaflets. They vary in style, and in the amount of detail they provide – ask to see some, and choose the ones which suit you.

The National Asthma and Respiratory Training Centre has produced a series of books specially written for parents and also for school teachers. In addition they have produced an asthma board game for children. All these items are available from the National Asthma and Respiratory Training Centre – the address is in the *Useful addresses* section of the Appendix.

Glossary

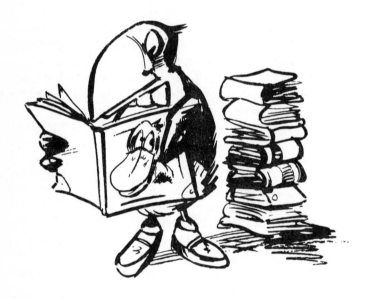

acute Short lasting. In medical terms this usually means lasting for hours or days, rather than for weeks or months.

adrenal glands Important glands in the body which produce a number of hormones to control the body systems. Cortisol and cortisone are two very important examples, and adrenaline is another.

airways When we breathe in and out, air has to travel through hundreds of branching tubes, or airways, to and from the lung tissue (see Figure 1.1). In asthma the problem lies with these airways, which become narrow, preventing air from moving freely in and out of the lungs.

allergens If you are 'allergic' to something, allergens are the tiny particles or substances to which you react when you come into contact with them.

allergic reaction This is what happens when you come into contact with something to which you are allergic. The allergic reaction varies from person to person and according to which part of your body reacts. For example, with grass pollen, an allergic reaction may take place in the lining of your nose (in which case you get hay fever); in the airways (causing asthma symptoms); or in the skin (causing urticaria, which is similar to nettle rash).

allergy To have an allergy means to overreact to something in a harmful way when you come into contact with it. If you have an allergy to grass pollen you will have streaming eyes and nose, and sneezing if you come into contact with it (hay fever). Someone who is not allergic to grass pollen will not even notice grass pollen when they are in contact with it.

alternative therapies Another name for **complementary therapies**.

alveoli These are the microscopic air spaces in the lungs which we refer to as the lung tissue. The airways get smaller and smaller as they divide into thousands of very tiny branches, and at the end of each of the smallest airways is an alveolus. It is in the alveoli that the air mixes with the bloodstream, and oxygen is taken in and carbon dioxide is passed out.

aminophylline Generic name for one of the reliever type of drugs. Aminophylline can be taken by mouth, or given by injection. There is no inhaled form.

anabolic steroids Anabolic steroids are **not** used in the treatment of asthma. They cause the body to build up muscle, and because of this have been taken by some athletes to improve performance and strength. They should not be confused with corticosteroids, which are used to treat asthma and a number of other medical conditions.

anti-inflammatory agents These are drugs which have an action against inflammation. Many diseases or conditions of the body – from asthma to arthritis or bowel disease – result in inflammation. Anti-inflammatory drugs reduce this inflammation and help the body to keep functioning as normal.

asthma register This is a list which is kept of people with asthma, usually by a general practice. All practices have a list of patients registered with them. A proportion of those will have asthma, and they are listed in a separate register. This has advantages, the most important of which is that the practice can organize its care for those with asthma, keeping a check on treatments, and how often to review people.

atopic or atopy To be 'atopic' is to have an allergic constitution. This means that in your make-up is the tendency to develop allergic, or atopic, conditions. The most important atopic conditions are hay fever and eczema. Asthma is strongly associated with atopy.

beta-2-agonists (also called beta stimulants or beta-2-stimulants) There are several names for this group of drugs, and this can be very confusing! Beta-2-agonists are the most important group of reliever drugs, and they include Ventolin and Bricanyl. Most often they are taken by the inhaled route, but also they can be given in tablet, medicine or injection form. Another group of beta agonists – the long-acting beta agonists – include the longer acting relievers salmeterol xinafoate (Serevent) and eformoterol fumarate (Foradil).

beta blockers These are very important drugs which may be used to treat high blood pressure, angina, anxiety, glaucoma and a number of other conditions. They have directly the opposite action to the beta agonists, so they are of no help to people with asthma, and can be dangerous. Nobody with asthma should take beta blockers, even in the form of eye drops, e.g. timolol, also known as Timoptol!

bone age As children grow, their bones grow with them (of course). As they grow, distinct changes can be traced in the bones by X-ray. If, for example, a child aged seven years has an X-ray of the wrist, certain changes can be seen which correspond to that age. In some children the bone age, as judged by X-rays, is ahead of or behind their actual age. This may be important in deciding whether a child's growth is being affected by a disease, or by certain drug treatments.

brand names All drugs in medicine have two names: their generic name, which is their true drug name; and a brand name under which they are sold by their manufacturer. For example, Aspro, Anadin and Disprin are all brand names of the drug aspirin.

breath-actuated device This is a type of inhaler device in which the drug is released only when a person breathes in. If no breath is taken, no drug is released from the device.

brittle asthma This is a severe variety of asthma and it is not very common. Anyone with asthma might suffer an attack which comes on very quickly. However, people with brittle asthma can change, within minutes, from having no symptoms at all to having a very severe attack, despite taking regular treatment. Their attacks can prove very resistant to treatment. People with brittle asthma often need repeated hospital admissions, and very intensive treatment.

bronchi and bronchioles Bronchi are the main branches of the breathing tube (respiratory) system, taking air in and out of the lungs (see **airways**). Each time they branch, the diameter of the airway becomes smaller. The very smallest branches of the system are called bronchioles, and they end in air spaces called alveoli.

bronchial hyperreactivity (also called bronchial hyperresponsiveness, BHR) This means an oversensitivity in the airways, so that when the airways come into contact with irritants (e.g. allergens, smoke, viruses) they overreact in a way which causes them to produce symptoms such as coughing and wheezing.

bronchiolitis An important chest infection which occurs in babies, usually in the winter months. It is caused by a virus, and often leaves the baby with coughing and wheezing for months or years afterwards.

bronchitis This is a very common chest infection. The main symptom is cough, with production of phlegm (sputum), usually yellow or green in colour. It may also cause wheezing and shortness of breath, and so can be confused with asthma. Acute bronchitis can occur in any age group at any time. Chronic bronchitis is a more serious condition of older people, usually smokers or those who have lived for years in polluted atmospheres.

bronchodilators A medical term for relievers. They are called bronchodilators because they open up (dilate) the airways (bronchi). There are three main groups of bronchodilators, of which the beta agonists (which include Ventolin and Bricanyl) are the most important.

candida infection Another name for **thrush**.

cardiac asthma This book is about **bronchial** asthma. Cardiac asthma is a different condition resulting from heart failure. In heart failure, fluid becomes trapped in the lungs because the heart cannot pump strongly enough to clear it. The symptoms include shortness of breath and wheezing, as with bronchial asthma, but their cause (and treatment) is completely different. Cardiac asthma is not a term which is used very often these days, which is just as well, since it can be confusing.

chronic In strictly medical terms, chronic means 'long lasting' or 'persistent'. In everyday use, many people using the word chronic mean severe or extreme. Both may apply. For example, chronic bronchitis by definition is persistent, but it often is severe.

complementary therapies Non-medical treatments which may be taken alongside conventional drug treatments. Alternative therapies is another term often used, but this suggests that the therapy is taken instead of rather than alongside conventional treatments. Popular complementary therapies include homoeopathy, acupuncture, osteo-pathy and chiropractic.

corticosteroids This is a group of chemicals produced naturally by the body (mainly in the adrenal glands) and also synthetically as drugs. They are vital for the body's own action against infection and stress; and in disease when given as drugs they are amongst the most effective and powerful agents available to doctors to treat inflammation. So, in asthma, which is a result of inflammation in the lining of the airways, they are the most effective treatment available.

cortisol or cortisone A corticosteroid produced naturally by the body, in the adrenal glands.

cyanosis A blue discoloration of the skin, lips and tongue which results from the blood carrying too little oxygen. In asthma attacks it is a sign of a very serious condition, and requires emergency treatment with oxygen.

danders (also called animal danders) Contents of animal hair, or fur, which cause an allergic reaction.

dehydration A condition in which the body is deficient in water. In asthma, this may occur over several hours, as a result of rapid breathing, vomiting, and difficulty in drinking usual amounts of fluid.

desensitizing treatments If you have a strong allergy to a single allergen, it **may** be possible to treat it with desensitization. This is a series of injections over several weeks. They contain gradually increasing strengths of the allergen. The theory is that the body can build up a gradual resistance in this way, and that this removes the allergy. In practice, desensitizing treatments may be effective; however, they are potentially dangerous. They are only used now in certain circumstances in specialist centres, for example for people with extreme bee sting allergy.

diurnal variation A change from one time of day to another 12 hours later, usually from early hours of the morning to evening. In this book we talk mainly about diurnal variation in peak expiratory flow readings, and this means the difference between readings taken first thing in the morning (which tend to be lower), and those taken in the evening (which tend to be higher).

dry powder devices Inhalers in which the drug is delivered in the form of a powder, rather than an aerosol spray. The main types of dry powder devices are Spinhalers (Figure 2.6), Rotahalers (Figure 2.2), Diskhalers (Figure 2.1), Accuhalers (Figure 2.7) and Turbohalers (Figure 2.8).

eczema (also called atopic eczema) This is a red, itchy inflammation of the skin, sometimes with blisters and weeping. There are several different types. Atopic eczema is common in children and is associated with other allergic conditions, particularly hay fever, and asthma.

exercise asthma Symptoms of asthma brought on after several minutes of exercise, particularly running. Exercise is one of the most important triggers of asthma symptoms.

extrinsic asthma Asthma which is clearly triggered by some external factor, particularly allergens such as house dust mite and animal hair.

generic names A general, or true, name for a drug. Different from the brand name which is given by the company that produces it. Any one drug can have several brand names but only one generic name.

genes A unit of heredity which helps to make up an individual's characteristics. Genes are contained on chromosomes in all the cells of the body. Each individual has his or her own set of millions of genes – half of which are inherited from the mother and half from the father.

hay fever A condition of the nose and eyes caused by allergy to grass pollen during the summer months of June and July. Sometimes the same allergy also results in asthma symptoms – so called 'pollen' asthma. Hay fever is also known as seasonal rhinitis.

house dust mite A microscopic insect, correct name *Dermatophagoides pteronyssinus*. It survives by feeding on dead scales of human skin. We all shed these in great numbers, continuously, and they collect in house dust, particularly in bedding. The house dust mite is the most important and common cause of allergy and allergic asthma in the UK. Numbers are high all the year round, but especially so in the early winter months.

hyperventilation Often known as overbreathing, this is breathing more often than the body needs for its oxygen requirements, and for getting rid of carbon dioxide. It occurs most often in periods of tension, anxiety or overexcitement.

immune system The body's own defences against outside 'attackers', whether they are infections, injuries, or other agents that are recognized as foreign, e.g. immunizations. The body's immune system reacts by attacking them, and producing antibodies which give more long-lasting protection against future attackers of the same type. For example, in an attack of measles, the body's immune system fights off the infection after several days, but also produces antibodies which will protect for many years against a future attack.

inflammation Inflammation is the reaction of the body to some injury, infection or disease process. Generally, its purpose is to protect the body against the spread of injury or infection. But in some cases, as in asthma, the inflammation becomes chronic, and this tends to damage the body rather than protect it.

intrinsic asthma Asthma which is not obviously triggered by any external agent, but tends to be continuous.

late onset asthma Asthma which begins in adult life, with no past history of it being a problem during childhood. Many people who appear to have late onset asthma will give a history of being 'chesty' children, or having repeated 'bronchitis' or 'pneumonia' as children. This suggests that their asthma is recurring in adulthood, rather than appearing for the first time.

late reaction When people with asthma are exposed to triggers for their asthma, they usually react within one hour, the 'early reaction'. However, there may be another 'late' reaction, which occurs approximately 6–10 hours afterwards. This is caused by a different set of reactions, but is every bit as important as the short-term reaction. Because of the time gap, it is more difficult to identify. It does not respond so well to reliever treatment as the short term reaction.

leukotriene receptor antagonists (LTRAs) These are new tablets that may be useful as preventers in the future management of asthma.

litres per minute The reading on the peak flow meter is measured in litres per minute. It refers to the number of litres per minute that would be blown out of the lungs if someone could continue at their peak expiratory flow.

long acting relievers The first long acting inhaled bronchodilator drug was called salmeterol (Serevent). Salmeterol xinafoate and eformoterol fumarate and the other bronchodilators have a long duration of action – around 12 hours – compared with around four hours for other relievers. Salmeterol xinafoate used to be referred to as a 'protector'. We now prefer to call it a 'long acting reliever'. It need only be taken twice daily.

lungs The organs of breathing. The function of the lungs is to take oxygen into the bloodstream, and to get rid of the waste product, carbon dioxide, into the exhaled air.

medical history Someone's past record of illnesses, symptoms and medical problems.

monilia infection Another name for **thrush** or infection with candida.

morning dip We all have a natural variation in our peak expiratory flow readings during day and night, which results in slightly lower readings in the morning than the evening. In asthma in general, and some people with asthma in particular, this pattern is very much exaggerated, so that a normal reading in the evening is followed by a pronounced 'dip' in the readings the following morning. This is recognized as an indication for changing treatment.

nasal polyp *see* polyp

NSAIDs (full name non-steroidal anti-inflammatory drugs) A class of drugs used extremely commonly for arthritis, other rheumatic conditions and generally for pain relief. Brufen or Nurofen (ibuprofen), Froben, Ponstan, Indocid (ibuprofen), indomethacin, Feldene and Voltarol are well known examples. All are related to aspirin, and in a few people can make asthma worse.

occupational asthma Asthma which results purely as a consequence of working in a particular environment. Important examples are given in the section on *Work* in Chapter 4. Proven occupational asthma is a prescribed disease, meaning that industrial compensation may be available if cause and effect can be proved.

oral steroids Corticosteroid treatment given by mouth. Nearly always this is given as prednisolone tablets.

osteoporosis Thinning of the bones which occurs as a result of overall loss of calcium from the body. The most important group affected by this is older women who lose bone density more rapidly after their menopause. The results of osteoporosis are an increased risk of fractures, particularly of the spine and thigh bone.

overbreathing Another name for **hyperventilation**.

ozone A gas, related to oxygen, which is present in small amounts in the atmosphere.

passive smoking Breathing in smoke from another person's cigarette, cigar or pipe.

peak flow In this book we refer to peak expiratory flow (PEF), readings, charts, diaries, meters and monitoring! A PEF is a very simple but effective measure of how hard someone can blow air out of their lungs. The instrument used to measure it is a peak flow meter. If the airways are wide open, then air can be blown out at a very high rate of litres per minute (l/min). If, as in asthma, the airways are narrowed down, then the PEF falls simply because air cannot be blown out at the same speed. A PEF reading is the measurement achieved on the scale of the meter; a peak flow chart is a record of PEF readings kept over a period of time, and a peak flow diary does the same, usually recording peak flow readings at particular times of day, and also keeping track of symptoms and treatment over the same time. Peak flow monitoring is usually carried out by the person with asthma. They have a home peak flow meter (available on NHS prescription) and can track their own condition, with assistance from their doctor or asthma nurse.

photochemical smog A very unhealthy atmosphere caused by a reaction between pollution near ground level and sunlight. This usually occurs in hot climates, where an urban environment is surrounded by mountains which tend to trap the air, e.g. in places such as Los Angeles and Athens. It has occurred in the UK, especially in London. The smog contains gases that are damaging to the lungs, and can make asthma very much worse. These are ozone, particulate matter and oxides of nitrogen.

pleurae Two layers of membrane which surround and cover the lungs internally as a protection. Infection of the pleurae results in pleurisy – a very painful condition.

polyp A small harmless growth which arises from an internal lining of part of the body, such as the lining of the bowel, or the nose. Polyps in the nose are quite common in adults with asthma, particularly those whose asthma started later in life. (People with polyps may be allergic to aspirin.)

prevalence The prevalence of a condition is the proportion of a population that has that condition. Prevalence may be current or cumulative. For example if we were to say that the current prevalence of asthma in the UK is 6%, we would mean that 6% of the population has asthma at the moment. We might also say that the cumulative prevalence is 30%, by which we would mean that 30% of the population have had asthma at some time in their life, but not necessarily at the moment.

preventers Drugs which are taken to prevent the symptoms of asthma from occurring, rather than to relieve them when they do occur. The most important group of preventers is the inhaled steroid drugs, described in Chapter 2.

prodromal (as in prodromal itching) Symptoms coming before the start of an illness or a condition.

propellants These include CFCs (chlorofluorocarbons) which are now banned because of their effect on the environment and HFAs (hydrofluoroalkanes) which have been developed to replace them.

protectors A term previously used to describe the first long acting reliever.

puffers A popular name for metered dose inhalers (MDIs – Figure 2.3). The most commonly used inhalers, which release a puff of spray containing the drug when the canister is pressed.

relievers The most frequently used type of anti-asthma drug. Relievers relax muscle spasm (tightness) around the airways, helping to open up the airways and relieve symptoms. Relievers are best used when needed rather than regularly. The most frequently prescribed reliever inhalers are Ventolin and Bricanyl. Reliever tablets and syrups – Bambec, Bricanyl, Phyllocontin, Uniphyllin, Ventolin and Volmax – are sometimes prescribed. *See also* long acting relievers.

remission A period of time without symptoms or problems from a condition. In asthma the most likely time for a remission to occur is in late childhood. Remission may last for many years, and treatment will not be required during this time. Asthma is such an unpredictable condition that it may go into remission at any time. However, the opposite also applies – after remission it may return at any time.

rhinitis Inflammation of the lining of the nose – similar to the process of asthma in the airways. In the UK the commonest reason for rhinitis is allergy to grass pollen (hay fever, or seasonal rhinitis). The symptoms of rhinitis are running of the nose, blocking, sneezing and itching.

rhinovirus A type of virus which is known to cause the common cold frequently, and in people with asthma to provoke episodes of asthma with a cold ('a cold going on to the chest'), especially during the autumn and early winter months.

season ticket Shorthand name for a prepayment certificate for NHS prescriptions. These may be purchased for three months or for a year. They are expensive, but if you require frequent prescriptions and are not exempt from charges you will probably save money by buying one. Pharmacists, Post Offices or Family Health Services Authorities will provide application forms.

skin prick tests Special tests to show whether a person has a tendency to allergy. Drops of solution containing allergen are placed on the forearm and the skin is pricked gently through the solution. A positive test occurs when a weal, like a nettle rash, appears within 10 minutes. The tests are painless and inexpensive. The results of these tests may provide helpful information for the GP or nurse.

steroids A particular group of chemicals which includes very important hormones, produced naturally by the body, and also many drugs used for a wide range of medical purposes. In asthma the subgroup of steroids with which we are concerned is the corticosteroids. Very often this term is shortened to steroids, causing people to confuse their asthma treatments with the anabolic steroids used for body building. Steroids provide two of the most important treatments for asthma: the tablet form (prednisolone) which is mainly used in short courses and can be a life saver in acute attacks; and the inhaled form which, as Aerobec, Becotide, Becloforte, Filair, Flixotide and Pulmicort, comprises the most important type of preventive treatment.

tartrazine An additive which formerly was found commonly in foods and soft drinks, but which increasingly is being removed. It is probably the most important food additive implicated in asthma.

theophylline Generic name for one of the reliever type of drugs. Theophylline can be taken by mouth, or given by injection. There is no inhaled form.

thrush (also called candida or monilia infection) A fungal infection of warm moist places in the body, particularly the mouth and skin folds. In asthma, thrush is an important side effect of inhaled corticosteroid treatment. It is also a frequent consequence of a course of antibiotic treatment. Usually it is easily treatable.

tidal breathing Breathing gently in and out at rest.

topical (inhaled) steroids Steroids which are inhaled or breathed in and so do not get absorbed directly into the bloodstream. This is an advantage, because it minimizes the risk of side effects. Inhaled topical steroids are used mainly in asthma (in inhaler devices) and in allergic rhinitis (e.g. hay fever).

trachea The main windpipe, which begins at the level of the voicebox, and goes into the top of the chest, where it divides into the bronchi (airways).

triggers Factors which **may** bring on symptoms or attacks of asthma. They do **not** cause asthma. Examples are given in the section on *Triggers* in Chapter 1.

twitchy airways An alternative name for **bronchial hyperreactivity**.

uncontrolled asthma The most important stage of asthma for you to recognize! This is when asthma begins to deteriorate, and heads towards an acute attack. If you can recognize it early, and take the right action, trouble will be avoided.

upper respiratory tract infection (URTI) An infection of the ears, nose and throat. The best known example is the common cold. Almost all URTIs are caused by viruses. This means they take their own time to disappear, and they are rarely helped by giving antibiotics, which do not have any effect on virus infections.

virus A microscopic organism, which multiplies in and attacks living cells, causing infections. There are many different groups of viruses and many thousands of different types of virus. The infections they cause vary enormously, from the trivial type to the fatal. Well known examples are the common cold, influenza, measles, hepatitis and AIDS. Virus infections are important in asthma because they are the commonest trigger for attacks. Colds going on to the chest, particularly in winter, are the triggers for many attacks. Virus infections are not helped by antibiotics.

Appendix

Useful addresses

Action Asthma Patient Service
Apartment 900
Freepost
Bradford
Yorkshire BD7 1BR
● Educational material for adults, teenagers and children

British Lung Foundation
78 Hatton Garden
London EC1N 8LD
Tel: (020) 7831 5831
Fax: (020) 7831 5832
Website: http://www.lunguk.org

Chest, Heart and Stroke Scotland
65 North Castle Street
Edinburgh EH2 3LT
Tel: (0131) 225 6963
Fax: (0131) 220 6313

Chest, Heart and Stroke
Association (Northern Ireland)
21 Dublin Road
Belfast BT2 7HB
Tel: (01232) 320184
Fax: (01232) 333487
Website: http://www.nichsa.com

Health Education Authority
Hamilton House
Mabledon Place
London WC1H 9TY
Tel: (020) 7383 3833

National Asthma Campaign
Providence House
Providence Place
London N1 0NT
Tel: (020) 7226 2260
Fax: (020) 7704 0740
● Educational material for health professionals and patients with asthma as well as their families, speakers for meetings, advice

- Telephone 'Asthma Helpline' 0845 701 0203. Weekdays 9.00am–7.00pm, calls charged at local rates from anywhere in the UK
- Local and self-help groups, social and fund-raising meetings
- Research
- The Junior Asthma Club

National Asthma and Respiratory Training Centre
The Athenaeum
10 Church Street
Warwick CV34 4AB
Tel: (01926) 493313
Fax: (01926) 493224
Website: http://www.nart.org.uk
- Courses on asthma for all health professionals
- Asthma clinic record cards for sale
- Schools Asthma Teaching Pack for Health Professionals
- Publications – *Asthma who cares? – A manual to help parents* and *Asthma who cares? – A recipe book to help with the management of asthma in schools*

Manufacturers

Advanced Allergy Technologies Ltd
Freepost ALM1541
187a Ashley Road
Hale
Cheshire WA15 9SQ
Tel: (0500) 004851
Fax: (0161) 929 6825
- Alprotec Allergen Exclusion System (mattress, duvet and pillowcase covers)

Allen & Hanburys Ltd
Stockley Park West
Uxbridge
Middlesex UB11 1BT
Tel: (020) 8990 9888
Fax: (020) 8990 4321
- Accuhaler
- Babyhaler
- Diskhaler
- Integra
- Metered dose inhaler
- Rotahaler
- Volumatic (spacer device)

AstraZeneca UK Ltd
Home Park Estate
Kings Langley
Herts WD4 8DH
Tel: (01923) 266191
Fax: (01923) 260431
- Metered dose inhaler
- Nebuhaler (spacer device)
- Turbohaler

AstraZeneca UK Ltd
King's Court
Water Lane
Wilmslow
Cheshire SK9 5AZ
Tel: (01625) 535999
Fax: (01625) 712457
● LRTAs

Aventis
50 Kingshill Avenue
Kingshill
West Malling
Kent ME19 4AH
Tel: (01732) 584000
Fax: (01732) 584080
● Metered dose inhaler
● Spinhaler

Boehringer Ingelheim Ltd
Ellesfield Avenue
Bracknell
Berkshire RG12 8YS
Tel: (01344) 424600
Fax: (01344) 741444
● Metered dose inhaler

Boots the Chemist
Brent Cross Shopping Centre
Hendon
NW4 3FB
Tel: 0181 202 5256
Fax: (020) 8202 9814
● Anti-allergy bedding covers
   (mattress, duvet and pillowcase
   covers)

Celltech Medeva Pharma Ltd
Medeva House
Regent Park
Kingston Road
Leatherhead
Surrey KT22 7PQ
Tel: (01372) 364000
Fax: (01372) 364018

Clement Clarke International Ltd
Edinburgh Way
Harlow
Essex CM20 2ED
Tel: (01279) 414969
Fax: (01279) 635232
● Mini-Wright peak flow meters
● Nebulizers
● Spirometers

Ferraris Medical Ltd
Aden Road
Enfield
Middlesex EN3 7SE
Tel: (020) 8805 9055
Fax: (020) 8805 9065
● Peak flow meters

Medic-Aid Ltd
Heath Place
Bognor Regis
West Sussex PO22 9SL
Tel: (01243) 840888
Fax: (01243) 846100
● Nebulizers

Napp Pharmaceuticals Ltd
Cambridge Science Park
Milton Road
Cambridge CB4 0GW
Tel: (01223) 424444
Fax: (01223) 424441
● Theophyllines

Norton Healthcare
Albert Basin
Armada Way
Royal Dock
London E16 2QJ
Tel: (01279) 426666
Fax: (08705) 020304
● Easi-Breathe

Novartis Pharmaceuticals
Frimley Business Park
Frimley
Camberley
Surrey GU16 5SG
Tel: (01276) 692255
Fax: (01276) 692508

3M Health Care Ltd
3M House
Morley Street
Loughborough
Leicestershire LE11 1EP
Tel: 01509 611611
Fax: (01509) 237288
● Autohaler
● Theophyllines
● Aerochamber

Vitalograph Ltd
Maids Moreton House
Buckingham MK18 1SW
Tel: (01280) 827110
Fax: (01280) 823302
● Vitalograph peak flow meters
● Spirometers

Index

Numbers in **bold** refer to the colour plates. All other numbers are page numbers. Those in *italics* refer to pages carrying illustrations; those followed by italic *g* refer to the glossary.

Have you found **Asthma at your fingertips** practical and useful? If so, you may be interested in other books from Class Publishing.

Allergies at your fingertips
Dr Joanne Clough £14.99
At last – sensible practical advice on allergies from an experienced medical expert.
'An excellent book which deserves to be on the bookshelf of every family.'
Dr Csaba Rusznak, Medical and Scientific Director, British Allergy Foundation

High blood pressure at your fingertips
NEW SECOND EDITION! £14.99
Dr Julian Tudor Hart with Dr Tom Fahey
The authors use all their years of experience as blood pressure experts to answer your questions on high blood pressure.
'Readable and comprehensive information.'
Dr Sylvia McLaughlan, Director General, The Stroke Association

Diabetes at your fingertips
£14.99
Professor Peter Sonksen, Dr Charles Fox and Sister Sue Judd
461 questions on diabetes are answered clearly and accurately – the ideal reference book for everyone with diabetes.
'I have no hesitation in commending this book.'
Sir Harry Secombe CBE, President of the British Diabetic Association

Stop that heart attack!
Dr Derrick Cutting £14.99
The easy, drug-free and medically accurate way to cut your risk of having a heart attack dramatically.
Even if you already have heart disease, you can halt and even reverse its progress by following Dr Cutting's simple steps. Don't be a victim – take action NOW!

Eczema and your child
Dr Tim Mitchell, Dr David Paige and Karen Spowart £11.99
This practical and medically accurate handbook will guide you through the maze of old wives' tales, unscientific advice and outdated treatments.
'It addresses the questions we are asked all the time.'
Mercy Jeyasingham, Director of Education and Information, National Eczema Society

Heart health at your fingertips
Dr Graham Jackson £14.99
This practical handbook, written by a leading cardiologist, answers all your questions about heart conditions.
'Contains the answers the doctor wishes he had given if only he'd had the time to think how best to put them.'
Dr Thomas Stuttaford, The Times

Psoriasis at your fingertips
NEW! £14.99
Dr Tim Mitchell and Rebecca Penzer
Packed full of practical information on the day-to-day management of psoriasis.
This essential manual helps you find out about the various treatments available, helping you to discover which work best for you, and giving you effective self-help routines.

Cancer information at your fingertips
£14.99
Val Speechley and Maxine Rosenfield
Recommended by the Cancer Research Campaign, this book provides straightforward and positive answers to all your questions about cancer.

Kidney failure explained
£14.99
Dr Andy Stein and Janet Wild
Everything you always wanted to know about kidney failure but were afraid to ask!

Parkinson's at your fingertips
NEW SECOND EDITION! £14.99
Dr Marie Oxtoby and Professor Adrian Williams
Full of practical help and advice for people with Parkinson's disease and their families. This book gives you the information and the confidence to tackle the challenges that PD presents.
'An unqualified success.'
Dr Andrew Lees, Consultant Neurologist, The National Hospital for Neurology and Neurosurgery

Stroke at your fingertips
NEW!
£14.99
Dr Anthony Rudd, Penny Irwin SRN and Bridget Penhale
This essential guidebook tells you all about strokes – most importantly how to recover from them.

It is full of practical advice, and includes recuperation plans; you will find this book invaluable.

Alzheimer's at your fingertips
Harry Cayton, Dr Nori Graham, Dr James Warner £14.99
At last – a book that tells you everything you need to know about Alzheimer's and other dementias.
'An invaluable contribution to understanding all forms of dementia.'
Dr Jonathan Miller CBE, President, Alzheimer s Disease Society

Epilepsy at your fingertips
Brian Chappell and Professor Pamela Crawford £14.99
The authors answer over 220 real questions from people with epilepsy – giving you the knowledge to lead an active and fulfilled life!

Multiple sclerosis at your fingertips
NEW! £14.99
Ian Robinson, Dr Stuart Neilson and Dr Frank Clifford Rose
The expert authors pass on all the useful, practical information they have learnt over the years. There is specific information on areas such as driving, holidays, work, children, sexual relationships and other people's attitudes
'An invaluable resource.'
Jan Hatch, Director of MS Services, MS Society

Your child's epilepsy: a parent's guide
£11.99
Dr Richard Appleton, Brian Chappell and Margaret Beirne
If your child has epilepsy, you will find this practical guide invaluable. It answers the questions you really want to ask from diagnosis to treatment, and from schools to relationships.

PRIORITY ORDER FORM

Cut out or photocopy this form and send it (post free in the UK) to:

Class Publishing Customer Service   Tel: 01752 202301
FREEPOST (PAM 6219)
PLYMOUTH PL6 7ZZ   Fax: 01752 202333

Please send me urgently (tick boxes below)   **Post included**
(UK only)   **price per copy**

☐	**Asthma at your fingertips** (ISBN 1 85959 006 3)	£17.99
☐	**Allergies at your fingertips** (ISBN 1 872362 52 4)	£17.99
☐	**High blood pressure at your fingertips** (ISBN 1 872362 81 8)	£17.99
☐	**Diabetes at your fingertips** (ISBN 1 872362 79 6)	£17.99
☐	**Stop that heart attack!** (ISBN 1 872362 85 0)	£17.99
☐	**Eczema and your child** (ISBN 1 872362 86 9)	£14.99
☐	**Heart health at your fingertips** (ISBN 1 872362 77 X)	£17.99
☐	**Psoriasis at your fingertips** (ISBN 1 872362 99 0)	£17.99
☐	**Cancer information at your fingertips** (ISBN 1 872362 56 7)	£17.99
☐	**Kidney failure explained** (ISBN 1 872362 90 7)	£17.99
☐	**Parkinson's at your fingertips** (ISBN 1 872362 96 6)	£17.99
☐	**Stroke at your fingertips** (ISBN 1 872362 98 2)	£17.99
☐	**Alzheimer's at your fingertips** (ISBN 1 872362 71 0)	£17.99
☐	**Epilepsy at your fingertips** (ISBN 1 872632 51 6)	£17.99
☐	**Multiple sclerosis at your fingertips** (ISBN 1 872362 94 X)	£17.99
☐	**Your child's epilepsy** (ISBN 1 872362 61 3)	£14.99

TOTAL: £_____

Easy ways to pay
Cheque: I enclose a cheque payable to Class Publishing for £_____
Credit card: please debit my ☐ Access ☐ Visa ☐ Amex ☐ Switch

Number: Expiry date: _____

Name _____

My address for delivery is _____

_____

Town   County   Postcode

Telephone number (in case of query) _____

Credit card billing address if different from above

_____

Town   County   Postcode

Class Publishing's guarantee: remember that if, for any reason, you are not satisfied with these books, we will refund all your money, without any questions asked. Prices and VAT rates may be altered for reasons beyond our control.

NATIONAL **ASTHMA** CAMPAIGN
conquering asthma

- Funds research into the causes and treatment of asthma.

- Gives help, advice and support to people with asthma, their families and carers.

- Provides education and information about asthma and its treatment.

- Has a network of local branches throughout the UK.

- Publishes a quarterly magazine for members.

- Funds an Asthma Helpline staffed by specialist asthma nurses.

- Offers support and information to all health professionals.

If you would like to become a member, or if you would like to send us a donation to support our work, then please fill in the form *overleaf* and return it to us at the address shown.

Guildford College
Learning Resource Centre

Please return on or before the last date shown
This item may be renewed by telephone unless overdue

- 6 JAN 2004		
- 8 JUN 2004		
2 9 NOV 2005		
2 1 FEB 2006		
2 2 MAR 2013		
1 4 APR 2015		

Class: _____ 616. 238 LEV

Title: _____ Asthma

Author: _____ LEVY, mark.

☐ what's happening in my local area
☐ the Junior Asthma Club for children aged 4–12 years

Send this form to: National Asthma Campaign, FREEPOST, London N1 2BR

THANK YOU FOR YOUR SUPPORT

Registered charity number 802364